Working with Traumatized Children

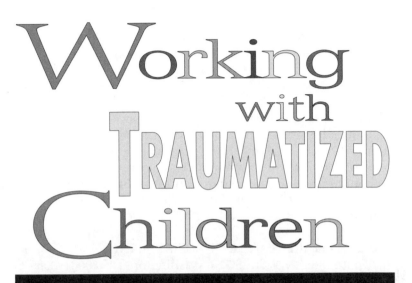

Working
with
TRAUMATIZED
Children

A Handbook for Healing

Kathryn Brohl

CWLA Press
Washington, DC

CWLA Press
is an imprint of the Child Welfare League of America, Inc.

CHILD WELFARE LEAGUE OF AMERICA, INC.
440 First Street, NW, Suite 310, Washington, DC 20001–2085
Email: books@cwla.org

CURRENT PRINTING (last digit)
10 9 8 7 6 5 4 3 2 1

Cover design by Jennifer Riggs–Geanakos
Text design by Jennifer M. Price

Printed in the United States of America

ISBN # 0–87868–633–9

Library of Congress Cataloging-in-Publication Data
Brohl, Kathryn.
    Working with traumatized children : a handbook for healing /
Kathryn Brohl.
        p.   cm.
    Includes bibliographical references.
    ISBN 0-87868-633-9 (pbk.)
    1. Post-traumatic stress disorder in children--Handbooks, manuals,
etc.   I. Title.
RJ506.P55B75   1996
618.92'8521--dc20   96-24093

This book is offered, with love, to every child care
professional who has made a commitment
to healing children.

It is also a tribute to those remarkable young people who
have encountered and survived traumatic experiences.

Lastly, it is dedicated to my daughter,
Susan Elizabeth Sharp,
and my very supportive husband, Phil Diaz.

∼ • *Contents* • ↗

⌐ • *Acknowledgments* • ⌐

In my training workshops, child care professionals have expressed a need for a practical handbook about trauma and children. Without their encouragement, this book would not have been written.

I also wish to acknowledge the unselfish sharing of the following people and agencies:

For typing sections of my manuscript, Sue Sereix.

For their ideas and suggestions, Scott W. Allen, Ph.D.; Ana Compo-Bowen, M.D.; Sal Fusaro, M.D.; Maria Iriate, LCSW; and Sandra Brookshire, Sarah Massey, Kathleen Hadeed, and Tammy Cross, from Dare County Department of Social Services in Manteo, North Carolina.

For inspiring several chapters, the staff at Vista Maria School in Dearborn, Michigan.

For being my patient mentor many years ago, Carol Brown, M.S.W., from Richland County Children Services, Mansfield, Ohio.

Finally, thank you to my husband, Phil Diaz, whose wisdom, encouragement, patience, support, and long hours spent helping me edit, particularly the resilience chapter, will always be appreciated.

✑ • *Introduction* • ✑

This practical handbook is designed to help you work with traumatized children. You may be a child protection, group home, addictions, residential treatment, rape, or domestic violence counselor. Or you may be a clinical social worker, psychologist, teacher, foster parent, or guardian ad litem volunteer. In the role of ancillary professional, you may be a police or probation officer, judge, attorney, or physician. Whatever your child advocacy job, guiding and/or treating traumatized children is an important mission.

This book is a reference and guide. It will help you understand how traumatic experiences affect children and what caregivers can do to foster the healing process from trauma. It also explains relevant treatment issues by describing the stages to recovery from trauma, panic attack intervention, and metaphorical storytelling. Additionally, it identifies some of the major resilience traits in children.

Finally, shaping children's lives is wonderful. It is essential to take time to appreciate what you do. Because so many adults have also been traumatized as children, I have provided a chapter for such caregivers and child advocates. This chapter highlights the strengths and liabilities caregivers who were traumatized as children bring to their work. It offers specific suggestions for the self-care of child advocates.

After a while, reading "she/he" can become tedious, so I have chosen to use the word "she" in referring to traumatized children and their helpers. The names of all children in this book have been changed to protect their privacy. Some information for the book was gathered through interviews; when not otherwise specified, interview settings are confidential.

∿ · *1* · ∿

Trauma and Its Impact on Society

Child advocates are becoming increasingly alarmed by the severity of abuse and neglect aimed toward children. Conventional interventions on behalf of young people are being re-examined. But reinventing social services for children is not easy. Contributing to the problem is the public debate on how money for youth can best be utilized.

Child welfare, however, is not an isolated problem and can not be resolved solely by dollars. Every sector of society must become involved, and public and private citizens must make a personal commitment to participate in the healing of youth.

Child advocates know that helping hurt children is not a simple task. It demands an understanding about the reasons children enter juvenile justice or child welfare systems. Most children within these systems have been traumatized. They often express abnormal and/or oppositional behaviors; characteristics associated with trauma. Without proper intervention and treatment, many children grow up to be even more troubled as adults.

Child care professionals need to understand the affects of traumatic experiences in children, in order to heal this problem and articulate its complexity to public officials and private citizens.

Dealing with Reality

The world is a changed and frightening place for children today. Incidents like the bombing of the federal building in Oklahoma City in 1995, which left 165 people dead, have contributed to the perception that the world is no longer a safe place. This perception has been compounded by a number of natural disasters such as the earthquakes in California, the floods in the Midwest, and the devastation left by Hurricane Andrew in South Florida. Many children were traumatized directly by those events; others were traumatized by witnessing the events or their aftermath on television. What is true of the world in general is reflected in the child welfare system.

Child welfare rules created during the 1970s have not kept pace with a changing world. A number of social issues have dramatically affected the child welfare system. According to the Child Welfare League of America, "alcohol and drug abuse are directly related to child and family well-being." For example, an infant exposed to alcohol and/or drugs prenatally is born every 90 seconds in the United States. Many of these children have learning or other developmental problems, and need expensive and exhausting care.[1]

Former Surgeon General Dr. Joycelyn Elders [1994] commented, "Many tough and complex public health issues involve some of the most private aspects of life." These private aspects of life include parenting children. Lack of effective parental involvement and clear societal norms have also influenced every socioeconomic group. As a result, our children have suffered.[2]

In Florida alone, kids have dropped one spot closer to the cellar. Second only to New York, Florida has more violent juvenile criminals than any other state—a 63% increase since 1985. Student drop-out rates in Louisiana and West Virginia have reached crisis proportions. These disturbing statistics are reflective of the child and youth conditions throughout the United States.[3]

The U.S. Advisory Board on Child Abuse and Neglect in 1995 released results from a two and half year study which included the following information:

- Abuse and neglect in the home is a leading cause of death for young children in the United States. Many abuses continue to go unreported. The majority of abused and neglected children are under four years old.

- Child abuse fatalities have risen 50% over the past eight years.

- An estimated 50% of homes with adult violence also involve child abuse or neglect.

- Many states lack adequate protections for abused children and legal sanctions for juvenile offenders.

- AIDS is threatening to become the leading adolescent killer in the twenty–first century. Fewer than half of sexually active teenagers reported using a condom in their last sexual encounter. Even fewer adolescents abstained from sexual contact at all.

- Nearly 30% of Americans under the age of 20 smoke cigarettes, and the average age for their first use is 11.5 years.

- About half of 18 to 20 year olds have used alcohol in the past month, and binge drinking has become a common form of recreation for young people in middle, senior high school, and college.

- About 40% of pregnant minority women do not receive any prenatal care in their first trimester.

- Violence is becoming the problem–solving alternative for many of today's youths. Gang crimes, as well as murders, acquaintance rapes, and drive-by shootings have increased.

- Children continue to have babies. With greater frequency, these babies are being abandoned physically, emotionally, and spiritually by their biological parents.[4]

Children continue to be on the losing side of poverty. The U.S. Department of Health and Human Services reported in 1996 that the percentage of children in "extreme poverty" (when the family income is less than half the official poverty level) has doubled since 1975. The poor living below the poverty line include one in every five children in the United States.[5]

These problems affect everyone. When care is poor, the ramifications for future generations are immense. Children will continue to suffer the effects of their poor caregiving long after they have grown to adulthood.

Douglas Nelson, executive director of the Annie E. Casey Foundation, states, "It may well be that the nation cannot survive—as a decent place to live, as a world class power or even as a democracy—with such high rates of children growing into adulthood unprepared to parent, unprepared to be productively employed, and unprepared to share in mainstream aspirations."[6]

Taking a Practical Approach

It has taken 25 years for the American public to understand the effects of the Vietnam war and the posttraumatic stress reactions in soldiers who fought there. The child welfare system is facing the same type of uphill battle as it tries to change society's approach to children who are fighting their way back from their own terrifying experiences.

Child care professionals work with children who have been traumatized by parental abandonment, abuse, or neglect. These youngsters fear for their physical or emotional integrity, and can become overwhelmed by their own physiological, emotional, and behavioral responses under stress. Their responses are similar to those demonstrated by Vietnam veterans. Other children who have experienced trauma in the form of natural disasters or the Oklahoma bombing can also be included.

This handbook takes a practical approach toward working with traumatized children. While providing a guide to understanding and treating trauma, it also emphasizes the *physiological* (or mind–body) connection to Posttraumatic Stress Disorder.

Caregivers can erroneously ignore the physical factors which contribute to a child's abnormal behaviors. When terrorized, children are affected to the extent that they remain susceptible to later feeling as though they are reexperiencing their trauma. Survival responses then emerge to fight against this terror and they develop numbing, avoidance, somatic, or any other number of maladaptive reactions.

This handbook also describes practical crisis intervention techniques. These interventions can provide immediate relief in children who experience panic.

Stacking the Deck in a Positive Direction

Understanding posttraumatic stress issues, and taking careful steps during a child's recovery, empowers the child care professional to successfully help the child transform disturbing maladaptive stress reactions and practice new coping strategies. Additionally, knowing more about trauma helps child care professionals convey the message to lay people and legislators about the answers to healing a troubled child.

Solving juvenile problems is complex. Many traumatized children have developed an extensive repertoire of destructive habitual responses to stress. Children can benefit or be cured with knowledge, team effort, and with firm, clear, loving, and consistent intervention. Children do recover from trauma.

Notes

1. Child Welfare League of America, *Children at the front: A different view of the war on alcohol and drugs* (Washington, DC: Author, 1992), p. 3.

2.   J. Elders, "Speak to the poor, the powerless," Farewell speech, *Miami Herald* (December 21, 1994), p. 25A.

3.   Annie E. Casey Foundation, *Kids count data book: State profiles of child well-being* (Baltimore, MD: Author, 1996).

4.   U.S. Advisory Board on Child Abuse and Neglect, *Child abuse becoming U.S. public health crisis* (Washington, DC: Author, 1995). J. Elders, "Speak to the poor, the powerless," Farewell speech, *Miami Herald* (December 21, 1994), p. 25A. Child Welfare League of America, *Children at the front: A different view of the war on alcohol and drugs* (Washington, DC: Author, 1992), p. 3.

5.   E. Gleick, "The children's crusade," *Time Magazine*, 147(23) (June 3, 1996), 30–35.

6.   *Ibid.*, p. 32.

~ • 2 • ~

Understanding Trauma and Posttraumatic Stress Disorder

Posttraumatic Stress Disorder (PTSD) is a relatively new medical diagnosis. Before 1970, it was largely considered by doctors to be a psychological rather than a physiological problem. Recent advances in research, however, confirm that PTSD is traced to a disruption in normal brain functioning.[1]

~ • *Mary Jo* • ~

Mary Jo* was four years old when she became trapped inside a discarded refrigerator laid to rest in a junkyard behind her house. She'd been drawn by her curiosity to unexplored territory. The ancient appliance provided a cool and quiet resting place.

Her peace was disrupted when she heard her grandmother's shrill voice calling to her. Sensing her grandmother's anger, Mary Jo closed the refrigerator door. She became terrified when it wouldn't open. Luckily, the owner of the junkyard came to her aid when he heard her muffled cries.

Following her rescue, Mary Jo had nightmares and began to cling to her grandmother when they separated.

---

* The names of all children have been changed to protect their identity.

7

Her stress was compounded when her father came to take her for short visits. Several times while bathing together, he hurt and terrified her as he inserted his finger into her vagina. (This behavior is referred to as digital penetration.)

Sadly, Mary Jo had no one to talk to about her traumatic experiences. Her mother had died; her grandmother was emotionally unavailable; and her father was sexually abusive. Mary Jo's family was ill-equipped to give her what she needed in the way of protective parenting.

At age 8, Mary Jo was removed from her grandmother's home and placed in out-of-home care. Nightmares, as well as her oppositional behavior, were noted upon her arrival. Her bed-wetting was noticed soon after.

Fortunately, Mary Jo was able to receive loving supervision and therapeutic intervention. Over time she was able to talk about her father and the terrifying experience in the refrigerator. Her physical and emotional problems eventually subsided.

Mary Jo's invisible wounds created abnormal behaviors typically exhibited by traumatized children. Other behaviors include the ones expressed in the following case examples.

⤙ • *Case Examples* • ⤚

Andy, age seven, is a withdrawn child with a history of bed-wetting and nightmares. He was physically abused by his biological father. Andy's mother is severely depressed and unable to care for her son. As a result, he was placed in foster care. Andy is becoming accustomed to his new surroundings, but his nightmares continue.

Jake watched while his sister shot her boyfriend. He expresses exaggerated startle responses and is excessively anxious. His father states, "Jake is 12. He's a big man now. The murder happened six months ago. He should get on with his life."

Stephanie's mother and brother were killed when they were on their way to pick her up at school. Stephanie, age 10, is severely depressed. She believes that she is to blame for their deaths and is being punished by God. Her grief-stricken father is barely managing to keep his remaining family members fed and sheltered.

Cory is a hyperactive nine-year-old, severely neglected by his mother. His anxiety and oppositional behavior try everyone's patience. He threatens and bullies other children. He has a difficult time earning small rewards at his residential cottage, and other children complain about his aggressiveness.

Sheree, a 15-year-old alcoholic, has been in three alcohol treatment centers, beginning at age 13. Sheree is an incest survivor who reports hearing voices. She says she drinks to "bring down their volume."

Traumatized children develop habitual stress responses such as explosive temper, sexualized behavior, flashbacks, nightmares, addictions, bed-wetting, and a host of other problems. Treating these particular "wounds" requires an understanding about how traumatic experiences create defensive reactions in children.

Posttraumatic Stress Disorder: The Mind-Body Connection

The old saying, "It's just in his head," is true when it comes to understanding Posttraumatic Stress Disorder. (It is also referred to as Posttraumatic Stress Syndrome.) Researchers believe that a terror experience can disrupt normal brain functioning.[2]

Following an inescapable (actual or perceived to be inescapable) catastrophic experience, a person's brain chemistry is altered, creating heightened sensitivity to adrenaline (also referred to as noradrenaline) surges. *Adrenaline/noradrenaline surges* cause human beings and other animals to become aroused in order to prepare to fight or flee from danger.

In a hypersensitive state, a person can be susceptible to noradrenaline surges long after being terrorized. In other words, one can remain vulnerable to feeling and reacting in fear when the initial terror is no longer present. A person is tricked by various stressors, into reacting as though she is still in danger.[3]

When stimulated to arousal, a person prepares for a fight or flight response to the imagined danger. A pounding heart, sweaty palms, headaches, loss of bowel or bladder control, an upset stomach, teariness, insensitivity to pain, and a host of other physical and psychological reactions can occur.

> Posttraumatic Stress Disorder is the emergence of characteristic symptoms that surface when a child's hyperaroused state causes her: to feel as though she is reexperiencing her trauma; and to persistently avoid any physical or emotional associations with the trauma.[4]

These symptoms are acquired as a result of a hypersensitive (aroused) condition. In this condition, a person is excessively sensitive to stressors which trigger an alarm for an emergency that is not there in reality.

More about Stressors/Triggers

Traumatized children are stimulated to arousal by a variety of stressors/triggers, or by physical and psychological associations with the traumatic experience. Stressors are personal. What triggers one child may not trigger another. Examples include:

- loud noises—yelling or cars backfiring;

- discussion about the trauma;

- feeling physically vulnerable—dressing out for gym, swimming;

- certain music, types of dancing, specific work of art;

- pressure to perform in a certain way;

- smells, textures;

- sexual contact;

- certain times of the day;

- certain anniversaries—rape, accident, birthday, death;

- developmental stages—entering first grade, puberty, leaving home;

- certain activities—bathing, visiting a doctor, driving;

- exposure to weapons—guns, knives, clubs; and

- certain physical characteristics—beards, long hair, old age.[5]

◣ • *Sarah* • ◢

During a birthday celebration, six-year-old Sarah believed she was reexperiencing a threat to her life when she saw the host use a knife to cut the cake. Even though she was currently living in a safe and supportive environment, she was triggered into believing she was reexperiencing her original trauma which occurred when Sarah witnessed her father slash her mother's face during a family celebration. The little girl responded to this "trigger" by becoming withdrawn, tearful, and clingy.

ie
later =
Page—16

Children like Sarah become hypersensitive. They may have yet to experience a moment when their bodies are calm rather than "alert." Ongoing hypervigilance is exhausting.

Learning new information is another challenge when the body becomes aroused. Often, the best that children can do, while controlling their internal fight or flight messages, is to remain quiet for a few minutes.

The state of experiencing paralyzing fear can also stop a child from speaking when she becomes triggered by a false danger signal. These states can overwhelm children and those who look after them.

Defining Trauma and Its PTSD Connection

DEFINITION

Webster's Dictionary [1990] defines trauma as "a disordered psychic or behavioral state resulting from mental or physical stress or physical injury," or "an agent, force or mechanism that causes trauma."[6]

Posttraumatic Stress Disorder arises *after* a child has experienced trauma. Symptoms usually appear around one to three months following the traumatic experience. Approximately half of the children diagnosed with PTSD recover after three months. Others, however, are affected much longer.[7]

Events which create PTSD include experiencing severe emotional and physical neglect; life–threatening situations such as murder or suicide; battering; sexual assault; ongoing screaming or verbal threats; certain physical separations from siblings or parents; and experiencing or being witness to wars, accidents, bombings, and/or natural catastrophes.

The American Psychiatric Association's Diagnostic and Statistical Manual of Mental Disorders IV [1994] states,

That a person (with Posttraumatic Stress Disorder) has been exposed to a traumatic event in which both of the following were present:
(1) the person experienced, witnessed, or was confronted with an event or events that involved actual or threatened death or serious injury, or threat to the physical integrity of self or others; and
(2) the person's response involved intense fear, helplessness and horror. Note: In children, this may

be expressed instead by disorganized or agitated behavior.[8]

An overwhelming feeling of being "trapped" is closely identified with PTSD trauma. Less severe stress, such as financial problems, does not create disruption in normal brain functioning.[9]

∿ • *Juanita* • ∿

Juanita is a child who was overpowered and terrorized when she was molested. At age five, Juanita's older brother forced her to engage in oral sex. Afterward, he warned her not to tell their mother. Juanita kept her traumatic experience to herself.

When she was six years old, her mother became ill and Juanita was temporarily placed in residential care. Upon her admission, child care workers noticed Juanita's lack of focus and short attention span. She was behind in school and became easily upset.

One evening, while playing with other children at her cottage, Juanita disclosed that her brother had put his "peter" in her mouth. When Juanita sensed her caregiver's interest, she became hysterical. After she was reassured that her brother would not return and hurt her, however, she calmed down.

Apparently, the security of Juanita's environment prompted the initial comment to her playmates. Over time, her ability to concentrate improved, and she became less easily upset.

Trauma Affects the Entire Physical System

Due to advances in brain photography/imaging, scientists are understanding more about what occurs within the brain when people are terrorized. Researchers, using Positron-Emitted Tomography (PET) scans, Electroencephalogram (EEG), or

---

Survival Response Systems

Limbic system—memory, learning, emotion

Endocrine system—metabolism, blood pressure

Autonomic nervous system—gastrointestinal

Immune system—thymus, spleen, lymph nodes, skin, etc.

Magnetic Resonance Imaging (MRI) can more accurately track brain activity.[10]

Scientists suggest that when someone is traumatized, chemical functioning within the brain becomes impaired, creating heightened sensitivity to becoming hyperreactive or hyperaroused. In this state, a trauma survivor is excessively sensitive to various stressors/triggers.[11]

Human beings and other animals have a lot in common, including shared survival responses. Wild animals spend a lot of time searching for their food, as well as desperately avoiding being food. In order to survive, they must be constantly alert to danger. Humans are also compelled to survive. Like the other animals, people with PTSD become hypersensitive to danger long after they have been traumatized.

Stressors/triggers (smells, visuals, emotional pressures, etc.) associated with the original trauma, register as danger to a trauma survivor. "Danger" signals activate the body into a fight or flight reaction. The alarm sends messages through the body to activate *survival response systems*. These systems are explained above. The activation of the Survival Response Systems can be

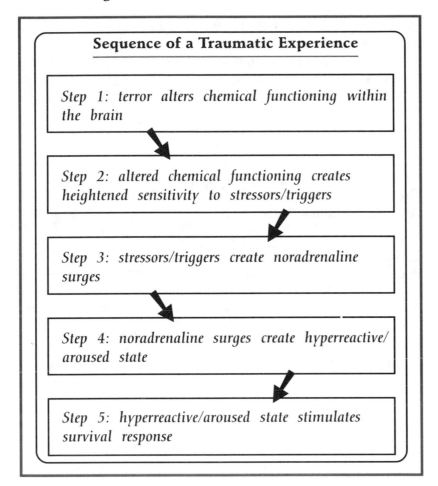

Sequence of a Traumatic Experience

Step 1: terror alters chemical functioning within the brain

Step 2: altered chemical functioning creates heightened sensitivity to stressors/triggers

Step 3: stressors/triggers create noradrenaline surges

Step 4: noradrenaline surges create hyperreactive/ aroused state

Step 5: hyperreactive/aroused state stimulates survival response

seen in children as: rapid heart rate, loss of bowel control, rashes, stomach aches, amnesia, dissociation, etc.[12]

The brain's information processing is disrupted during a terror experience, causing numbing to occur. Psychological or physical pain associated with the trauma can be blunted. For example, memories of the trauma can become distorted or completely forgotten. Other types of dissociation, or protective distancing is expressed through daydreaming, inability to concentrate, excessive tolerance for physical pain, and in extreme cases, multiple personality disorder. The sequence of a traumatic experience is diagramed above.[13]

One way to understand the mind–body connection and trauma is to try the exercise on page 17.

Stressor/triggers stimulate the child to react as though she is still in the midst of her initial trauma. Using the previous example of Sarah's experience at the birthday party, her condition begins and escalates like this:

Trigger .... *knife*
Memory-Picture .... *father-mother*
Threatened State .... *terror*
Physical/Emotional Response .... *heart/breathing*
                                                                     clinging/crying

Factors Affecting PTSD

The severity of stress responses in trauma survivors can be influenced by these factors.

(1)   Factor: Stress experienced *before* traumatic experience

Children who sustain long–term stress are predisposed to developing PTSD. After Hurricane Andrew in 1992, PTSD emerged more severely in young survivors if they had already been in accidents, or experienced disruptive moves.[14]

(2)   Factor: Caregiver support following traumatic experience

Family environment impacts on how a child interprets her traumatic experience. The quality of emotional support and appropriate problem–solving skills demonstrated by caregivers can positively or negatively influence a child's reaction to trauma. Discussing a traumatic experience, for example, quickens her recovery; whereas suppressing discussion of her experience impedes it.

Try This Exercise

Close your eyes. Mentally identify a traumatic memory. Bring to mind a picture of that event. As you are recalling your experience, you may begin to notice changes within your body. Your heart rate increases or you experience one of those distressing stomach knots. You may feel a lump in your throat. Notice any emotions. Take a deep breath and open your eyes.

The sequence of responses, looks like this:

Memory　➜　**Threatened State**　➜　**Physical/**
(or other stressor)　　　　　　　　　　　　**Emotional Response**

During this exercise, did your physical and emotional responses appear with the memory picture? Triggers can create rapid-fire reactions within our bodies. (This explains why we often observe dramatic changes in children.)

Recording Your Responses

When people record this exercise they become more enlightened about the mind-body connection to terror experiences. On another sheet of paper, record your recognitions in the format shown below.

My Memory　➜　**My Fear**　➜　**My Physical/**
(or other stressor)　　　　　　　　　　　　**Emotional Response**

➤ • *Allison* • ➤

Allison was 12 when an older neighbor boy entered her home and raped her while her parents were away. Allison, believing she caused her rape, kept the experience to herself. Her observant mother, however, noticed that Allison was unusually withdrawn. She gently questioned her daughter about her different behavior. Tentatively, Allison disclosed the truth. Her parents proceeded to file a police report and make counseling inquiries.

Allison's path to recovery was made smoother with family support. It meant the difference between her healthy recovery or acquiring long–term PTSD symptoms. Sadly, not all traumatized children are as fortunate. Another child's family may be excessively angry and/or depressed. She may have little opportunity to discuss her experience.

Children often mimic family coping styles or conditions in an attempt to overcome their trauma. Negative generational coping styles include using excessive drugs, alcohol, or expressing other types of numbing behaviors. On the other hand, if caregivers are emotionally supportive and role model appropriate coping skills, young survivors will draw upon these familial impressions, in order to process their experience in more productive ways. (Chapter Seven will discuss resilience factors.)

(3)   Factor: Ongoing stress *after* the traumatic experience

Trauma may not immediately create posttraumatic stress symptoms in children. Later losses such as the departure of a consistent caregiver may trigger the posttraumatic stress reactions in children who earlier appeared unaffected. (Note: Not everyone, including children, acquires PTSD following a traumatic experience.)

Understanding the Invisible Wounds

Understanding how a trauma experience can create Posttraumatic Stress Disorder is necessary when working with traumatized children. It is also useful to know that these children are
not usually "making up" their moods and behaviors. There is a
physiological link between a terror experience and the body's
adaptation to that experience.

We can help children understand that their bodies and
minds may react to a perceived threat, but, in fact, they are not
in danger *now*. When children integrate this message, they
begin to feel safe, their bodies are taken off "alert," and their
minds are open to learning new information. By viewing trauma
through this awareness window, caregivers can be more objec-
tive and knowledgeable when they guide young people
toward recovery.

Chapter Three will discuss stress responses in traumatized
children. Other chapters will outline child–specific interventions that reframe trauma impressions and heal self-
destructive stress reactions within children.

Notes

1.   K. Peterson, M. Prout, & R. Schwarz, *Posttraumatic stress disorder: A
     clinician's guide* (New York: Plenum Press, 1991).

2.   D. Goleman, "Key to posttraumatic stress lies in brain chemistry,
     scientists find," *New York Times* (June 12, 1991), Health section.

3.   *Ibid.*

4.   American Psychiatric Association, *Diagnostic and statistical manual of
     mental disorders, IV* (Washington, DC: Author, 1994).

5.   K. Brohl, *Pockets of craziness: Examining suspected incest* (New York:
     Lexington Books, 1991).

6.   *Webster's Ninth New Collegiate Dictionary* (New York: Merriam Webster,
     1990).

7.   American Psychiatric Association, *Diagnostic and statistical manual of
     mental disorders, IV* (Washington, DC: Author, 1994), pp. 424–429.

8.   *Ibid.,* p. 428.

9. D. Goleman, "Key to posttraumatic stress lies in brain chemistry, scientists find," *New York Times* (June 12, 1991), Health section.

10. S. Vandantum, "Brain scans aid doctors in diagnosis, in treatment," *Miami Herald* (May 13, 1996), p. 6A.

11. D. Goleman, "Key to posttraumatic stress lies in brain chemistry, scientists find," *New York Times* (June 12, 1991), Health section.

12. E. L. Rossi, *Pyschobiology of mind-body healing: New concepts of therapeutic hypnosis* (New York: W. W. Norton, 1986), pp. 27–39.

13. D. Goleman, "Key to posttraumatic stress lies in brain chemistry, scientists find," *New York Times* (June 12, 1991), Health section.

14. F. Shapiro, *Eye movement desensitization training*, Speech at EMDR Certification Training, New York (November 4, 1994).

～ · 3 · ～

Recognizing PTSD Symptoms

Children Develop a Variety of PTSD Symptoms

Following a traumatic experience, children may develop a wide range of adaptive responses in order to cope with their arousal states. *Adaptive responses (or reactions)* are defense mechanisms which emerge to guard against experiencing the original physical or psychological pain associated with their trauma. Several adaptive reactions will be discussed in this chapter.

Rage

Rage is often present in traumatized children. An excessive anger expression, it is a primitive survival response, generated by the brain's limbic system. Expressions of rage include suicidal or homicidal ideation and explosive temper. When older children combine rage with drugs or alcohol, the results can be disastrous. Younger children express their rage through aggressive play and exaggerated tantrums.

Excessive Aggression

An aroused child, responding to false danger messages, may become *excessively aggressive*. For example, one way children show aggression is to physically and verbally lash out at parents, siblings, peers, teachers, counselors, or other caregivers. It is often expressed by children in residential facilities. Destroying property, kicking furniture, and rough and sometimes violent play are familiar aggression scenarios at treatment centers. Even very young children may become excessively aggressive fol- lowing a traumatic experience. This true story drives home a powerful message.

❦ • Jimmy • ❧

Beginning in his infancy and ending at 15 months, little Jimmy witnessed his father beat his mother. His father was eventually incarcerated, and after release from prison, was court ordered to remain away from Jimmy and his mother. He was, however, allowed to speak by phone with Jimmy, now age three.

After Jimmy and his dad began phone contact, day care workers noticed that the little boy became aggressive with the other children. At the day care center, Jimmy's aggressiveness was reported to emerge within minutes after speaking to his father. His PTSD symptoms also escalated at home. He often hit his mother and cried out angrily in his sleep. Once his baby-sitter reported that while Jimmy slept, he shouted, "No Daddy, no hit Mommy!"

Jimmy's mother engaged a therapist who worked with small children on trauma issues. The effects of having witnessed his father batter his mother were particularly noted during one therapy session when Jimmy, without prior discussion about his dad, blurted out, "My Daddy hit my Mommy's back." Immediately Jimmy's face became contorted and he growled. His small hands clawed the air. Following this surprising disclosure, he sighed deeply and laid down on a cushion.

Prior to this session Jimmy had never referred to his father's battering. Later, his mother confirmed the episode in which he witnessed his father hit her on the back. (Note: Jimmy's mother did not fit a profile for parents who coach their children into false memories.)[1] ☆ *Reference*

Jimmy's agitated state was expressed through his aggressiveness. His symptoms subsided over time with play therapy and cessation of phone contact with his father. (His therapist believes that his father's voice may have stimulated Jimmy's hyperaroused state.)

Examples of excessive aggression include children who kill other children. These incidents occur too frequently. Robert was an 11-year-old child gang member in Chicago who murdered a 14-year-old girl. In retaliation, warring gang members murdered Robert. Ironically, the young boy was buried with his teddy bear.

Depression

Depression is a mood disorder and is often described as the condition of directing homicidal feelings toward oneself. It develops when children feel helpless to verbalize or otherwise be outwardly expressive. Feelings of being unable to control the anger and sadness related to their trauma are present.

Additionally, children are naturally self-centered. Consequently, they often believe that they were in some way responsible for, or could have prevented, their traumatic experience. They assume responsibility for what occurred, adding guilt and shame to their repertoire of feelings.

There are numerous ways in which children express depression. More pronounced examples are flat facial expression, excessive crying, severe mood swings, suicidal behaviors or ideation, withdrawing from previously gratifying hobbies or play, eating disorders, or general listlessness. Many times depressive disorder dovetails with other PTSD symptoms; however, depression is a dominant mood associated with PTSD. ☆☆

Numbing

The brain's adaptation to trauma includes *numbing* or *blunting*. One reaction tied to numbing is self-mutilation. This adaptation is particularly frightening in children. Caregivers often feel helpless and frustrated when they notice a child's self–inflicted tattoos, cuts, and burns. It can be difficult for them to understand that this adaptation emerges to defend against feeling panic and brings momentary relief to the self–mutilator.

Self–mutilation is just one example of numbing. An article in *the Washington Post* discusses *repressed memory*, another adaptation. The article states that a videotape was found by a junkyard employee in a car about to be demolished. The tape showed scenes of a man involved in sexual acts with a little girl. Fortunately, the name of the child's mother had been written on the outside of the tape.[2]

When contacted, the mother stated she had been unaware of her six year old's molestation. Social Workers who interviewed the child, now age nine, determined that she did not remember the incident. While none of the acts involved intercourse with the child, there was enough sexual contact demonstrated on the tape to prosecute her abuser.

This article leads one to wonder what caused the child to forget her experience. One answer proposes that during her molestation she had been triggered into a survival reaction, creating dissociative amnesia.

Repression of memories is confirmed in a study by University of New Hampshire sociologist Linda Williams. She interviewed 200 women taken to a hospital for child sexual abuse in the 1970s. But 17 years later, 38% did not remember or report the episode. Fifteen percent of those who did remember, said they had forgotten about it at one point.[3]

This next story illustrates how repressed memory affects someone while they sleep.

❤ • *Tasha* • ❤

Tasha was raped at age 13 in her own home. While her parents were out of town, her 16-year-old sister gave a party. An acquaintance came into Tasha's bedroom.

The 20-year-old assailant was much stronger than Tasha and horribly cruel. He tore off her panties and raped her. Eventually, a friend of her sister's forced open the bedroom door and disrupted Tasha's suffering. Her rapist disappeared. Tasha was terribly shaken and bruised, but she asked her rescuer not to mention the rape to anyone. She later recalled that she immediately took a shower and then phoned a girl friend, so that she could spend the night.

Tasha did not tell anyone about her rape. Like many children, she felt ashamed, embarrassed, and guilty. The morning following her vicious assault, Tasha helped her sister clean the house. The next day she went to school. Her traumatic experience became a dim memory.

Tasha soon began to express rebellious behavior. Additionally, she stopped wearing dresses, and her family complained that she was uncharacteristically sullen and withdrawn. For years she fought with her parents, and later, she dropped out of college. Her resilient coping adaptation was dancing. Tasha had gotten involved with this activity shortly after she'd been traumatized. Later, this outlet became a career. But unfortunately, her moodiness and intense panic feelings, which emerged when she was alone, did not subside.

At age 28, Tasha fell in love with a terminally ill man. After his death, she began waking up at night in small pools of her own blood. She had taken a sharp object while asleep and had cut herself. Tasha was shaken, horrified, and confused.

Later when she was questioned by her mother, Tasha spontaneously remembered her rape. She and her mother connected this memory to her self-mutilation. Following her disclosure, Tasha was positive that she would no longer hurt herself while she slept.

Sadly, this did not happen. Tasha continued to awaken with her arms slashed; once requiring stitches. Finally,

Tasha sought the help of a therapist who was able to help her reprocess her rape and identify the terrified 13-year-old within herself. Happily, this young choreographer no longer experiences these episodes.

Other Numbing Behaviors

Tasha's story illustrates what can happen when the blunting or numbing function of the brain becomes activated. Other ways people numb themselves to dissociate from feeling retraumatized include:

- fugue (sudden, unexpected travel away from home or one's usual place of work, with inability to recall the experience);[4]

- feeling separate from one's body;

- excessive fantasizing and magical thinking;

- lack of concentration to the point of not noticing physical obstacles;

- high-risk play which includes jumping off roofs, fascination with fire or matches, and endangering others while playing;

- auditory hallucinations which include hearing unexplained noises such as crying or screaming;

- visual hallucinations such as seeing ghostlike figures near the bed upon waking or falling asleep;

- attention-deficit;

- short or long term memory loss;

- compulsive behaviors, such as repetitious hand-washing or organizing;

- multiple personality infusion (the development of separate personalities within the child or adolescent);

- developmental regression, such as thumb sucking, baby talk, or separation anxiety; and

- time–learning confusion.[5]

Panic Attacks and Avoidance Behaviors

Panic attacks occur when children, in hyperaroused conditions, reexperience terror feelings. It is difficult for an adult to be articulate when she is panicked. Think of how overwhelming it must feel to a child, who because of her age, is intellectually less developed.

Many stressors/triggers ignite panic attacks, and often they seem harmless; for example, watching a television talk show on abuse, or even meeting someone new. Panic attacks occur within children when they take baths, visit relatives, attend a new school, or dress out for gym.

Avoidance behaviors emerge as conscious or unconscious attempts to avoid stressors/triggers which stimulate panic. Some of these avoidance behaviors can lead to drug use. These behaviors include glue sniffing, smoking marijuana and cigarettes, taking Xtasy or LSD, snorting cocaine, and drinking alcohol.

Other avoidance behaviors include being preoccupied with criticism or social rejection, developing phobias to sensory or physical reminders of the trauma, excessive caution with regard to trying new experiences or projects, and avoidance of school or other outside group activities. Children with PTSD avoid situations to the extent that it seriously impairs their ability to maintain and progress in their physical and psychological development.

✦ • *Janet* • ✦

Ten-year-old Janet avoided going to school following a traumatic experience when she had entered her home alone and happened upon two burglars. Although they did not physically hurt Janet before their escape, they threatened to return and harm her. The episode left her feeling dazed and frightened.

A few months following the incident, she began to avoid going to school; unusual behavior for Janet. Apparently, her avoidance behavior emerged when she imagined returning home after school. Janet's anxiety was related to her fear that she would be surprised and overwhelmed again.

Distrust

"When I see it, I'll believe it" is a stance taken by many traumatized children. Traumatic events often occur unexpectedly, surprising and confusing young victims. For example, anticipated vacations are ruined by a terrible car accident, or a long-lost family member returns to sexually molest his niece. Poor psychological support dovetails with these traumatic experiences; causing children to become *distrusting* and overly cautious.

High-Risk Behavior

High-risk behaviors are frequently connected to other PTSD symptoms, often masking anxiety and/or depression. This symptom threatens the physical or emotional integrity of a child or others. It is sometimes referred to as *passive suicide*.

One example of high-risk behavior is oppositional behavior, such as disregarding authority to the extent that it places a person at risk for incarceration. Other behaviors, such as sexual promiscuity, threaten physical health.

Children display high-risk behavior when they play in traffic, challenge angry people, carelessly handle guns, and participate in physical activities without proper safety equipment.

◆ • *David* • ◆

David lived in a residential treatment center for adolescents. He'd been in residential care for the majority of his 14 years because his mother was able to care for him *only when she did not have a boyfriend. David suffered from neglect, yet continued to idealize his mother. He frequently ran away from his placements to be with her.*

His high-risk behaviors were first noticed when he was identified as the seven-year-old "caped" child jumping off the roof of his foster parents' garage. David was redirected toward less risky distractions, but the boy seemed compelled to place himself in physically dangerous situations.

After years of work, staff members at his center felt that David's high-risk behaviors were diminishing. One weekend, however, his mother failed to appear for a visit. David shrugged off his disappointment. He later ventured outside to teach younger residents to fly kites. He had been warned to stay away from power lines again and again, but unfortunately, the warnings went unheeded. Sadly, his kite tangled with a power line and David was electrocuted.

David's tragedy reminds us that high–risk behavior causes senseless and untimely death in children. Working with risk-taking youths means working with children who consistently test their boundaries.

Testing boundaries is an attempt to master anxiety and depression. It is helpful for caregivers to remember that safety is the major consideration for traumatized children who are easily triggered into experiencing a hyperaroused state.

Sexualized Behaviors

Overt, compulsive, and unusual *sexual behaviors* in children can be conditioned responses to previous abuse and/or a habitual reactions to anxiety. Some of these behaviors in traumatized children include persistent masturbating in public places, molesting other children, using objects as sexual stimulants, sexual promiscuity, unsafe sexual practices leading to early pregnancy and sexually transmitted diseases, sexual play with animals, and exhibiting sexually provocative behaviors.

Sexualized behaviors in children are most often noticed and reported in residential treatment facilities, foster homes, schools, or other institutions. One child care professional in Florida said, "I wouldn't have believed it if I hadn't seen it. One moment Jackie was playing nicely with his little brother and the next Jackie's hand was in his brother's pants." These incidents happen quickly, and often, during play.

Less than 20 years ago children were frequently blamed when they were sexually molested; especially when a child, exhibiting sexually provocative behaviors, disclosed she had been molested by a family member. A classic example is that of a five-year-old child who was fondled by her father. When the case was being investigated, I overheard a sheriff's deputy saying, "That kid acts like she wants it." *Hopefully, these attitudes have changed.*

Flashbacks

The human brain is like a computer as it records and processes information. When trauma occurs, normal brain functioning is impaired, so that recollection of the event, along with sensory association with the event (visuals, sounds, smells) may be stored. *Flashbacks* in traumatized children are the memories of traumatic experiences that resurface.

Stressors/triggers can stimulate trauma memories and/or sensory recall to create flashbacks. People feel as though they are reexperiencing their trauma. Flashbacks have been described as bad "virtual reality" experiences. For example, pictures, noises, and smells associated with the traumatic experience may be spontaneously brought to the conscious mind. Children often feel terror in response to these pockets of surfaced recollections, believing the trauma is happening again. (Vietnam veterans have been courageous in speaking about their flashbacks since the war. Their information has assisted researchers in learning more about PTSD.)

Child trauma survivors experience flashbacks, creating greater problems for children because they lack the communication skills to articulate what is happening to them. As a result, they may feel isolated and misunderstood. Caregivers can become confused about what is really happening when a child launches into a temper tantrum or suddenly disappears out a window.

Sleep Disturbances

Trauma can disrupt normal sleep patterns. Frequently, young trauma survivors experience the same nightmare for years. Fear of reexperiencing these dreams can later lead to insomnia and exaggerated reactions to sleeping alone.

Sleep disturbances can be linked with avoidance behaviors and other posttrauma defense mechanisms, and include sleep-walking, excessive sleeping, the inability to experience a certain level of sleep, such as the rapid–eye–movement (REM) stage, deep sleep stage, or twilight sleep. Sleep deprivation and/ or sleep disturbances can severely affect youngsters, to the extent their ability to handle stressors and process information becomes impaired.

Obsessive-Compulsive Adaptations

Children with *obsessive-compulsive adaptations* to trauma attempt to gain mastery over their anxiety by paying attention to sched-ules, rules, and orderliness. These children repeat behaviors and often check for mistakes. Adolescents who become involved in activities such as high school ROTC often channel compulsive behaviors in a positive way. Other obsessive–compulsive characteristics are hoarding objects, inflexibility, rigidity, and displaying exaggerated behaviors when disappointed.

Somatic Complaints

Experts suggest that a child's physical system may be weak-ened during and following a traumatic experience. Trauma-tized children may more easily acquire infections, digestive problems, rashes, double vision, and/or paralysis or localized weakness. Headaches, dizziness, loss of balance, unexplained choking, and breathing disorders are other *somatic responses* to trauma that disrupt normal routines and impair learning.[6]

One little girl in foster care believed she was going to die from the same disease that took her mother's life. In fact, she registered an abnormal blood count. Thoroughly examined, it was clear she had not acquired her mother's illness. The low blood count persisted, however. As she felt safer in her new surroundings, it spontaneously became normal.

Eating Disorders

Eating disorders are often traced to traumatic experiences. *Anorexia nervosa* is the refusal to maintain a normal body weight. *Bulimia nervosa* involves binge eating followed by purging behavior such as self-induced vomiting, use of laxatives, excessive exercise, and fasting. These behaviors develop in latency age and adolescent children. Eating disorders emerge to avoid feeling overwhelmed by terror feelings related to their trauma and to gain personal control.

Elimination Disorders

Elimination disorders are also examples of PTSD symptoms. They include *encopresis*, or passing feces in inappropriate places, and *enuresis*, or the repeated voiding of urine into bed or clothes. *Constipation*, another elimination disorder, is the inability to pass feces. (Many times the cure for constipation, enemas or taking mineral oil, can seem traumatic to children.)

Suicide and Suicidal Ideation

Feelings of hopelessness are often present in children, who have been traumatized. Children, like adults, are susceptible to feeling worn down by life's obstacles. Despair can lead a child to fantasize about *suicide* or to actually commit suicide.

Additionally, children experience survivor's guilt similar to the guilt expressed by Holocaust survivors. For example, guilt feelings in children can be caused by being spared while other passengers have died in an auto accident or by outliving close relatives. "Why didn't God take me?" or "Did they die because I was bad?" are statements made by young survivors of trauma. Survivor's guilt may lead to suicidal thinking.[7]

Caregivers must be alert to early warning signals. Journals, poetry, and artwork are barometers of suicidal ideation and provide windows of opportunity to intervene in behalf of a child. Additionally, helpers must be willing to go the extra mile for a child who is vulnerable to suicide. A list of warning signals is provided on page 34.

Stress Adaptations Are Seldom Seen Alone

Common sense dictates that a child does not have PTSD because she has a bad temper. Posttraumatic Stress Disorder is defined by more than one symptom. Most PTSD symptoms dovetail with one another. For example:

Jerry—explosive temper, stomach problems, school phobic

Natalie—rashes, nightmares, depression

Tony—aggressive, academically challenged, impulsive

Kisha—mute, enuresis, obsessive–compulsive

PTSD Inhibits Normal Development

Posttraumatic Stress Disorder symptoms can inhibit a child's normal growth and development and cause considerable suffering. When children become distracted, their learning suffers. Additionally, when they avoid fear–inducing situations, they may not be able to master developmental stages, such as forming relationships and separating from home. Ironically, other stress adaptations build character and foster resiliency. Those responses will be discussed in Chapter Seven.

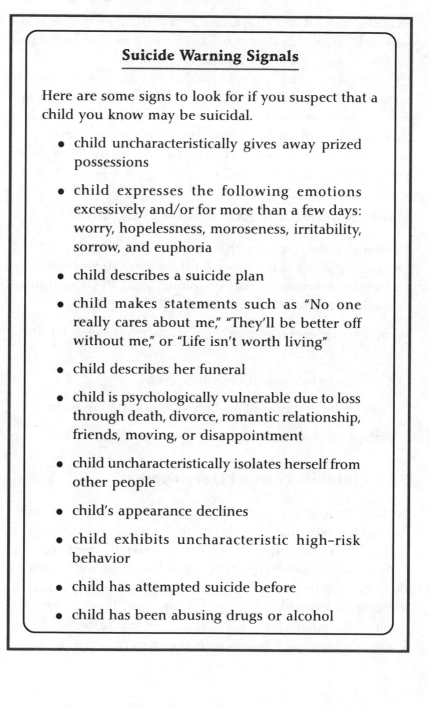

Suicide Warning Signals

Here are some signs to look for if you suspect that a child you know may be suicidal.

- child uncharacteristically gives away prized possessions

- child expresses the following emotions excessively and/or for more than a few days: worry, hopelessness, moroseness, irritability, sorrow, and euphoria

- child describes a suicide plan

- child makes statements such as "No one really cares about me," "They'll be better off without me," or "Life isn't worth living"

- child describes her funeral

- child is psychologically vulnerable due to loss through death, divorce, romantic relationship, friends, moving, or disappointment

- child uncharacteristically isolates herself from other people

- child's appearance declines

- child exhibits uncharacteristic high–risk behavior

- child has attempted suicide before

- child has been abusing drugs or alcohol

Notes

1. R. Gardner, *The parental alienation syndrome and the differentiation between fabricated and genuine sex abuse* (Cresskill, NJ: Creative Therapeutics, 1987).

2. A. Lester-Thomas, "Fresh evidence in a junkyard: Video-tape leads to trail of child abuse," *Washington Post* (October 18, 1990), p. C1.

3. B. Rubiner, "Memories serve in court," *U.S.A. Today* (November 29, 1993), p. A2.

4. American Psychiatric Association, *Diagnostic and statistical manual of mental disorders, IV* (Washington, DC: Author, 1994), p. 484.

5. K. Brohl–Hagans, & J. Case, *When your child has been molested: A parents' guide to healing and recovery* (New York: Lexington Books–MacMillan International, 1988). C. Peterson, M. Prout, & R. Schwarz, *Post-traumatic stress disorder: A clinician's guide* (New York: Plenum Publishing, 1991).

6. M. J. Horowitz, *Stress response syndromes* (2nd ed.) (New York: Jason Aronson, 1986).

7. M. E. P. Seligman, & S. T. Maier, "Failure to escape from traumatic shock," *Journal of Experimental Psychology*, 72(1) (1967), 1–9.

~ • 4 • ~

The Recovery Process

Recovery Stages and Intervention Goals

Working with traumatized children requires knowing the PTSD recovery process. It is summarized in this chapter, with an understanding that an entire volume may not exhaustively cover this subject. Knowledge of these stages provides necessary background information for discussion of intervention strategies in later chapters.

There are three stages in trauma recovery; a beginning, middle, and end. They are referred to as the *confusion*, *reorganization*, and *integration* stages. Specific intervention goals apply to each stage. The stages and goals are outlined on page 38.

Stage One: Confusion

Helpers become acquainted with a traumatized child during the confusion stage, when PTSD symptoms have escalated out of control. A child may have begun outpatient counseling or have been placed in out-of-home care.

These children are in crisis; their PTSD symptoms seem overwhelming. They feel powerless to control their fears, which are easily triggered, and they struggle to feel safe. They may be distrusting of new helpers or the helpers' intentions.

Stages and Goals of Recovery

Confusion Stage

(1)   Helper forms an emotional attachment with child.

(2)   Helper reassures child that her trauma is not happening right now.

(3)   Helper reassures child that she (the child) is not responsible for her trauma.

(4)   Helper reinforces positive changes in child.

Reorganization Stage

(1)   Helper asks child to notice how her body:
   • feels when the child is feeling safe; and
   • feels when the child is feeling unsafe.

(2)   Helper asks child to notice what causes the child to feel unsafe.

(3)   Helper guides child through her unsafe moments.

(4)   Helper reinforces positive changes in child.

Integration Stage

(1)   Helper engages child in deeper discussion about her trauma.

(2)   Helper teaches child new coping skills.

(3)   Helper facilitates child's resolution of her trauma.

(4)   Helper reinforces positive changes in child.

GOALS: One of the goals in the first stage is to psychologically connect with a traumatized child. Caregivers can establish a relationship in a variety of ways. Some of them include:

- skillfully listening;

- participating in an activity *with* children; and

- paying special attention to a birthday or accomplish-ment.

Forming attachments to others can intimidate traumatized children. But creating a safe relationship with a child lays the foundation for proceeding through the recovery process.

Another goal is to reassure children that the original trauma is not reoccurring. In fact, the chances of experiencing the exact traumatic event again are very slim.

Finally helpers must drive home the message that children are not responsible for their trauma and are not bad people because they experienced trauma. One way to accomplish this goal is to encourage children to verbalize or otherwise notice their feelings of guilt or shame.

Stage Two: Reorganization

In Stage Two, PTSD symptoms occur less often and with less intensity. Youths become more aware that stressors can trigger false danger signals throughout their bodies. Children also begin to identify their particular stressors. During this stage they are guided through hyperaroused moments. Additionally, they are forming positive relationships with and beginning to seek help from others.

GOALS: Goals in Stage Two include reassuring children they are safe and asking them to notice *when* they feel safe. Children are also taught to discriminate between "safe" and "unsafe" situations. And helpers ask them to identify their stressors or triggers.

Guiding children through their hyperaroused states is an important goal. When children panic, helpers can

CM
panic

follow the three steps outlined below to alleviate the panic
feelings.

(1) Reassure children about their current safety status. (They
are safe *now*.)

(2) Reassure children that their panic feelings will pass.

(3) Explain and demonstrate exercises to cope with panic
feelings. (Examples include: deep breathing, journaling,
physical exercise, drinking cold water, listening to sooth-
ing music, or contacting a support person.)

Stage Three: Integration

In Stage Three, children have a clearer understanding that they
were not responsible for their traumatic experience. Self-
esteem increases as they become aware that they are not "bad"
because something bad happened to them. Additionally, as they
overcome their panic moments and practice new coping skills,
their anxiety diminishes. PTSD symptoms can disappear or
diminish as children apply these new recognitions.

GOALS: Helpers support in–depth discussion about the previous traumatic experiences. Changed behavior is rewarded when
helpers reinforce positive relationships, provide rewards, or plan
for family reconciliations.

Caregivers will begin to teach more sophisticated problem-
solving and coping skills, such as budget planning and hypothetical thinking about the future. Finally, professionals will
help children to resolve their trauma by assisting with con-
frontation or resolution sessions or helping children to separate from home.

EXAMPLE: Ronnie's PTSD recovery occurred over years as it
progressed through the three stages. This young man had been
physically abused by both parents and placed in foster care at
age 14. Though very intelligent, he performed poorly in school.
He also suffered from severe bouts with depression.

Shortly after his placement, Ronnie was evaluated medi-
cally and psychologically. A treatment team, which included
his foster parents, caseworker, and a psychiatrist, developed a
plan for his recovery. The team wanted to see if other interventions would be effective before he was prescribed an antide-
pressant medication.

The plan was successful. Ronnie responded without the
introduction of medicine. (Note: Many times children need the
help provided through medication. A psychiatrist is the most
qualified professional to make a medication decision.) Ronnie's
recovery is described within his story.

~ • *Ronnie* • ~

*When Ronnie came to live with his foster parents, he
was shy and withdrawn. It took him a while to warm
up to his new surroundings. Ronnie gradually became
attached to his foster family after several successful family
outings and as his foster mother became involved at
his school. He also formed relationships with his
caseworker and therapist, who he saw on a weekly
basis.*

*With the help of his support team, he was able
to understand his depression. He learned to identify
what caused him to become frightened or sad. Over
time, he was taught how to work through his unsettling
feelings by practicing stress releasing exercises. And when
his feelings threatened to overwhelm him, he asked for
help.*

*With encouragement, he became involved in track
and developed an interest in writing. His confidence
grew when he received awards in these activities. Ronnie's
self-esteem improved to the point that he even participated
in his school's peer counseling program.*

*As he neared his high school graduation, Ronnie
expressed deep concern about his future. A planning*

session was scheduled with his foster parents, biological parents, and support team to discuss his plans. After discussing his options after graduation, Ronnie decided to enroll in college.

Now, at age 21, Ronnie is a full-time college student. He visits with his foster and biological families, and checks in for therapy as needed.

The Puddle Story

Recovering from Posttraumatic Stress Disorder is analogous to a story about a man who walked through a puddle.

Once upon a time, a man walked through a puddle on his way to work. During the night, it rained and the puddle grew bigger. The following day, he walked through the same puddle. This time the man noticed that walking through the puddle made his feet wet and ruined his shoes. The next day, he walked around the puddle and when he got to work, he studied a map. Being very smart, he knew what to do. The following morning, he traveled a different road to work; thereafter never needing to sidestep a puddle.

Other Considerations

Healing from a traumatic experience can take hours or years, depending on a number of factors. These factors, included in Chapter Two, range from the severity of the trauma to how children are supported afterward.

From time to time, children may need to pay special attention to their stressors. Therapy is often reintroduced as children enter new developmental stages. For example, sexually abused children may be triggered into a hyperaroused condition when falling in love. But the positive message is that aroused states generally diminish in intensity and occur farther apart. Caregivers must be truthful with children and let them know that listening to their stressors is a lifelong exercise.

✒ • *Gina* • ✒

Gina, now 23, had been traumatized in first grade when she was molested by her uncle. Successful therapeutic intervention helped her process her experience. Later, when Gina grew older and became sexually active, she again needed help. Another intervention helped her understand her confusing and frightening responses to making love. Gina is now able to enjoy a sexual relationship with her fiancé.

Clear Guidance Is Needed

Children are looking for clear, strong guidance from caregivers. Understanding PTSD recovery stages and goals places helpers on solid ground and gives children direction as they heal from their trauma.

∼ • 5 • ∼

Healing Interventions

Approaches to Working with Traumatized Children

Through the years, various treatment strategies have been successfully utilized with traumatized children. Some of them include: cognitive–behavioral therapy, gestalt therapy, hypnosis, psychodrama, and group counseling. These methods have brought about positive results when a relationship has been established between a helper and a young person. Little treatment can occur, however, until a child's "safety" issues are addressed.

Well–meaning caregivers may attempt to elicit information about a trauma before a child feels secure sharing it. Ill–timed discussion can create long–term adverse effects in a child. Discussion without discretion can cause a youth's fears to surface, leading her to experience a fight or flight response. If she feels threatened, frank discussion can impede her recovery process. (Note: Child advocates, such as child abuse investigators, police officers, attorneys, and judges, will gather additional information by applying this knowledge in their interviews with children.)

Consequently, in order to proceed with further discussion, caregivers must:

[handwritten margin note: Safety Issues #1 priority]

- help children to feel safe (provide a safe environment);

- reassure children they are not reexperiencing their trauma; and

- begin to help children identify what triggers their hyperalert state (identify stressors).

Helping Children Feel Safe

Children feel safe when they know there is no present danger which will violate their physical or emotional integrity. Children feel safe when they understand guidelines or rules. They also feel safe or reassured when they receive positive feedback. Additionally, firm, clear, loving, and consistent validating helps children feel safe. Reassuring children is easy when they are calm, but it can be challenging when they are hyperaroused.

When children become aroused, their PTSD symptoms can create havoc. Yet during these unsettling moments, children must continue to be reassured. They need to be told that their former traumas are not reoccurring. For example, when children are out of control and placed in a "time-out" space, they can be told they are safe within that space. Comments such as, "No one can hurt you while you are here," or "Your behavior tells me that you don't feel safe. Feeling safe is a calmer feeling," can be effective.

If a child is being physically restrained, the professional can continue to reassure her that she is safe by saying, "Right now, you are being held because you are out of control. Your fear causes your body to hurt yourself or someone else. I want you to notice that you can change the fear. When you feel safer, I won't restrain you." Repeat this message again and again. After a time, she will begin to connect with the idea that fear creates her hyperalert condition.

Chapter Two described how children become sensitive to danger after they have been traumatized. Different settings, people, or routines can stimulate heightened awareness. For this reason, it is important to keep an observant eye on children who are newly admitted to a hospital or school.

Safety Checklist

Compiling a list of questions which addresses a child's safety issues can prevent hyperreactive states and provide valuable treatment information. The Safety Checklist on pages 48–49 becomes a reference for caregivers and can be integrated into treatment planning.

It is not always possible to ask or to receive answers to the questions. But helpers need to make an attempt to elicit information about a child's past and present safety concerns as soon as possible.

Questions can be asked in a variety of ways. Professionals can ask questions while helping a child unpack, making a bed, or while playing basketball together. They can be asked anywhere, and any time a genuine answer may possibly be received. One child care worker reported that she received her most meaningful information when she completed a chore activity *with* a youth.

Another way to acquire information is through play therapy, such as using art, puppetry, or psychodrama. Older children respond to writing exercises done with their nondominant hand or to keeping a journal.

Asking questions from the Safety Checklist in the early stages of a relationship with a child provides the helper with important information. And these same questions may be asked later in order for the helper to gauge the child's recovery progress.

Intervening with a Hyperaroused Child

When a child is falsely triggered into a panic attack, *the goal is to diffuse or dissipate her terror as soon as possible.* When the fear subsides, her symptoms diminish as well.

Safety Checklist

Ask these questions when you think you will receive the truest answers. Record them for future reference.

- Do you feel safe right now? (this moment)
- What makes you feel safe? (certain people, objects, etc.)
- What do you keep with you that makes you feel safe or loved? (teddy bear, pillow or blanket, locket, pictures)
- What makes you nervous? (loud noises, school work, pressure)
- How can I help you feel safe?
- What frightens you?
- What is your favorite thing to do?
- Does anything frighten you at night?
- Does anything frighten you about being *here* (when child is in residence) at night?
- Is there anyone working here, who makes you feel safe?
- What do you do when you feel scared?

- Is there anyone here who frightens you?
- Do you notice any changes within your body when you become frightened? (heart rate, upset stomach, headache, etc.)
- How would your life be different if you felt really safe?
- What causes you to become angry? (or sad, happy, depressed, etc.)
- What do you think will happen to you when you become frightened?
- What do you think about most of the time?
- Is there anyone who you fear will hurt you right now?
- Does anyone here remind you of someone who hurt you before?
- What do you do when you become disappointed?
- Do you ever tell yourself that you're a bad person?
- What do you say to yourself about who you are when you are sad or disappointed? (This is an important question that bears repeating.)
- Would you like to say something different about yourself when you become sad or disappointed?

Children assume these survival states automatically and at the most inopportune moments. As a result, child care professionals are often called at inconvenient hours or find themselves in the middle of a shopping mall with a panicky child.

Intervention Part I

The first part of the intervention describes how to calm a child, help her identify what triggered her behavior, and help her to notice her physiological state.

(1)   The helper makes sure the child is safe *right now*. She interrupts the behavior that is causing the child harm and checks out the child's physical well–being. If a child is calling from a phone booth late at night, she is asked to let the helper know where it is and if she's been harmed. The helper stops a physical or verbal fight, separates a child from another caregiver, or places a child in a safe space.

(2)   The helper asks the child to describe a picture of what happened when she was triggered into her aroused state, by saying, "Let me get the picture about what happened *within* you just now."

(3)   The caregiver repeats exactly what she hears the child report. For example, "Let me see if I have the picture." Then she repeats the *exact* information back to the child. DO NOT INTERPRET. If the child says, "I got in the car," the caregiver says, "You got in the car." (This type of *exacting* repetition diffuses emotion and creates connection.)

(4)   The professional gets an agreement from the child that what she heard her say was correct. If the child does not agree, the professional reports back to the child until the child agrees on what she reported.

(5) The young person is asked to give feedback about what she may be feeling within her body, in terms of uncomfortable sensations, such as a rapid heart rate, headache, sweating, nausea, stomach pains, lump in the throat, breathing problems, etc.... The helper says to the child, "What do you notice in your body right now?" or, "Does any part of your body feel upset?" After receiving each report from the child, the helper says something encouraging like "Good," "I get the picture," "Yes," and so forth.

(6) If the child is truly not in danger *now*, the caregiver lets her know she is not in danger. (She is usually not in danger now.) For example, the caregiver says, "Look around you *now*," "Notice, that you are not being attacked," "The good news here is, you're not in danger right *now*," or "I realized something great, you're not in danger *now*, the way you were before," and "You may think the rape is happening now, but it isn't, and that's a really helpful thing to know."

Intervention I Dialogue

SCENE: *Child care professional,* SANDY, *is called into the bedroom by* TANYA's *roommate, who states that* TANYA, *age 10, has been destroying the roommate's property.*

(1)* SANDY *interrupts* TANYA's *destructive behavior and does what is necessary to place* TANYA *in a safe setting. The safe setting may be* TANYA's *bedroom, a counselor's office, a time-out space, or the cottage living room.*

(2) (SANDY *gets the picture of what happened from* TANYA.)
SANDY: Tanya, I want to get a picture of what just happened. I want to know.
TANYA: I'm going to beat his ass.

---

* Numbers in dialogue correspond to the stages previously listed.

(3)   (SANDY repeats.)
       SANDY: You're going to beat his ass.
       TANYA: Huh, uh. That no good for nothing little piss ant.
       SANDY: That no good for nothing little piss ant.
       TANYA: He's telling me all this crap.
       SANDY: He's telling you all this crap.
       TANYA: He tells me that my daddy's going to jail.

(4)   (SANDY *gets an agreement from* TANYA *about the picture.*)
       SANDY: Let me get this picture. I want you to tell me if
            this is right. You're going to beat your roommate's
            ass. You think she's a piss ant, cause she told you all
            this crap about your daddy going to jail.
       TANYA: No, not my roommate.
       SANDY: Who, then?
       TANYA: My therapist.

(5)   (*After repeating the picture again, this time including the infor-
       mation about the therapist, not the roommate,* TANYA *agrees that*
       SANDY *has the picture.* SANDY *asks* TANYA *to notice any physical
       reactions.*)
       SANDY: Good. You were clear about that. Did you notice
            your body getting mad when he said that?
       TANYA: I don't know what you're saying.
       SANDY: Well, sometimes our bodies help us to know we're
            upset. What your therapist said may have felt scary
            to you, and your body got the message to fight.
            When you think about all of this, do you notice
            your heart beating faster, or do you want to cry? I
            notice that you've made a fist with your hands.
       TANYA: Yeah. My face is hot... I want to smash him with
            my fists.

(6)   (SANDY *asks* TANYA *to notice if her body is responding to fear
       now.*)
       SANDY: Is your body as mad now, as it was when you

were tearing up your roommate's pictures?

TANYA: Kinda.

SANDY: Right now, do you think your body is as afraid
or mad as it was before?

TANYA: I'm still mad, but not as mad.

SANDY: If the number 10 were the most mad and number 1 were the least mad, what number mad are
you now?

TANYA: About five.

SANDY: Wow, you've noticed something about your
anger and your body and you've noticed that your
feelings and body can change.

The caregiver should STOP here if unable to process the panic
attack or other reaction any further. Many times, it's enough to
stop the survival response. However, if there is time and the
traumatized child appears responsive, the caregiver can proceed to step 7.

Intervention Part II

In the second part of the intervention, the child is asked to
become more aware about her fears and how they impact
behavior. Additionally, alternative ways to cope with fear are
suggested.

(7) The helper asks the child what happened right before
her panic attack was triggered and her symptoms surfaced. She is asked for a picture again. For example, "Tell
me what you remember you were doing, or what crossed
your mind, right before you had the: flashback, threw
up, ran away, struck your teacher, etc...."

(8) The helper reports back to the child what she stated;
"Let me see if I have the picture right," and then repeats
the *exact* report. Again, DO NOT INTERPRET.

(9)   The child is asked if there had been anything about the event or situation that may have caused her to become frightened. (If she is unable to make a connection between the event and a fear, it is okay. You are carefully asking her to confront those things which frighten her into an aroused state.) Whatever answer the child gives, the helper responds by saying, "Yes," "Okay," "Good," or "Fine," "I see," "Got it," etc.

(10) The fight or flight episode is reframed for the child. For example, the helper says, "When you were in this kind of situation *before*, you would panic. Now, you know you're not in danger, but you can still feel the fear within your body. You even know that what scared you caused you to want to fight somebody. Then, guess what? Your body reacted and you started throwing things," or, to use another example, "When you were in this situation before, you've gotten scared and you would binge. Now, even though you may feel scared sometimes, you know you don't have to binge." Helpers should remember to make connection statements, so that the child can "connect" the fear to the behavior, while understanding she is not in danger *now*.

Intervention II Dialogue

(7)* (SANDY *asks the child to recall what happened before she felt upset within her body.*)

SANDY: Tanya, before you got mad, tell me what happened?

TANYA: What?

SANDY: Well, you agreed your body felt different. What happened before it changed? Did it become upset when your therapist told you about your dad, or right before you ripped up your roommate's pictures?

---

* Numbers in dialogue correspond to the stages previously listed.

TANYA: I saw Jeff, my therapist, and he said, "Did I know my dad couldn't visit me cause he was in jail?" Like I'm stupid.

(8)   (*Again,* SANDY *repeats the picture and gets agreement.*)
SANDY: Jeff asked you if you knew your dad was in jail?
TANYA: Yeah.

(9)   (*Eventually,* TANYA *discloses that she felt angry when she got back to her room.* SANDY *repeats this information and* TANYA *agrees.* SANDY *inquires if the experience frightened* TANYA.)
SANDY: Did you feel scared when you thought about your dad in jail?
TANYA: No.
SANDY: Is it scary to think you could be alone?
TANYA: Yes.
SANDY: I'm glad you told me this. Do you think that when you thought about your dad going to jail, you got scared to be alone? When you got scared, you re-acted by becoming angry (mad) and you hurt someone's things?
TANYA: Yeah.
SANDY: This is a good thing to know when you get scared, because a part of you knew it doesn't help you to hurt someone or their things. What can you do in-stead of taking your anger out on yourself? (SANDY *explains how people can continue to hurt themselves long after they have been hurt by someone else. At this time, she may insert a metaphorical story, outlined in Chapter Six.*)

(10)   (SANDY *reframes the episode, inserting coping alternatives to* TANYA's *fears.*)
SANDY: So, when you heard about your dad, you got scared, and then mad, and then you tore up your roommate's stuff. This is very helpful information,

because now when you get scared, you can let me know and I can let you know you're going to be okay and you don't have to hurt anything. Some of the ways blank *(insert the name of the child's favorite celebrity)* gets his anger out are to hit his pillow or tear up his old newspapers. I also know that he runs to get that energy out. Next time you're angry, I'll help you get your anger out so it doesn't hurt you or anyone else.

Helpers can utilize the Safety Checklist on pages 48–49 during the intervention. Information, such as knowing that calling a friend, talking to a child care worker, hugging a favorite pillow, or hearing a metaphorical story calms a child, can be incorporated into the intervention. It allows personal coping suggestions to be inserted into the conversation.

The child is always reminded that scary feelings, or any negative feelings, *pass*. One way this is done is by describing feelings as passing clouds. Helpers reassure the child that her fears *do* pass!

After completing Intervention I or II, the fact that the child/adolescent lived through her episode of fear is emphasized. The child is congratulated for:

- contacting a helper or coach;

- recognizing her defensive responses;

- any awareness she gained about self-nurturing; or

- acknowledging that she's not in danger *now*.

Finally, she is redirected toward a safe activity or helped to resume her normal routine.

Over time, repeating these interventions teaches a child to transform her survival responses. Additionally, when a helper consistently refers to her successes in getting past those fear messages, her resiliency skills are reinforced.

Reminders

Entering through a back door to gently calm a frightened child is preferable to entering through a front door with a fog horn. As the caregiver asks safety and other awareness questions, while reaffirming present reality, children are gradually able to recognize and change their PTSD symptoms.

Caregivers should remember that it can be a mistake to agree with a child that she is experiencing her original trauma again. In other words, while it is understandable for a helper to slip and speak of past traumas in the present tense, doing so can reinforce the child's belief that it (the trauma) is ongoing.

Getting the picture, making connections, reassuring about safety, and finally reframing the trauma creates successful change in children. Helpers need to keep in mind three important factors.

(1)   When reframing the PTSD episode, a child's PTSD adaptations are described in the past tense.

(2)   When reframing the child's fear, a new and more truthful message about a child's current danger situation is inserted, such as "The good news is you're safe now." It is important to remember PTSD is related to situations which occurred in the past.

(3)   The child is helped to pay attention to the fact that her arousal messages are often false alarms.

Chapter Six discusses a less intrusive intervention technique, metaphorical storytelling. This approach is an effective way to help children confront their fears while they reprocess their traumatic experience.

∽ • 6 • ∾

Metaphorical Storytelling

Storytelling is an ancient form of communication. In more recent times, folk tales have proved valuable in teaching morality and problem solving to children. The story of *Sleeping Beauty* speaks to emotional awakenings, and *Jack and the Beanstalk* describes a hero's escape from an adversary.

Metaphorical storytelling is a valuable psychotherapeutic aid. Symbolic representations of life's conflicts, struggles, and solutions described within stories are nonthreatening ways to communicate with traumatized children. Sigmund Freud, C. G. Jung, and Milton Erickson were well known psychiatrists who successfully used metaphorical storytelling in their work. Other professionals, such as teachers, child care workers, and attorneys, can also be effective storytellers.

ie therapist use storytelling

The metaphorical story *Baby Lamb and His Father* was written to assist six–year–old Ryan cope with his father's alcoholism. After hearing this story, Ryan began to sleep in his own bedroom, resume his normal eating habits, and verbalize his anger about his father's drinking.

∽ • *Baby Lamb and His Father* • ∾

Not long ago, Baby Lamb was born in a beautiful meadow. He lived with his mother and played with other little lambs. One day his mother said, "It is time

59

*that we visit your father." The little lamb was happy
to follow his mother down the path toward his father's
house.*

*As they walked, the sky grew dark and it began
to rain. The little lamb shivered as the wind blew stronger
and the air turned cold. When they arrived at his father's
home, the baby's mother said, "It has been a long
time and you don't remember your father, but he is
eager to see you." She knocked on the door.*

*It was opened by a very large ram. When he peered
down at his son, he frightened the lamb. The baby
noticed that his dad seemed strange. In fact, the baby
noticed he did not seem like other sheep. His father
swayed from side to side and smelled funny.*

*Suddenly his father began to shout at Baby Lamb's
mother. "Why haven't you brought my son to see me
before? Look at him! He looks just like me! I could
have taught him all kinds of things by now!" The
baby's mother calmly responded, saying "The baby has
always been with me. You could have seen him anytime
you wanted. I know you've been drinking poison water
again. I will bring the baby back another day." His
mother nudged Baby Lamb and they turned back to
their beautiful meadow.*

*Baby Lamb cried all the way home and was unable
to eat his dinner. Later he couldn't sleep. He was confused
and frightened. Baby Lamb thought that he had done
something wrong to cause his father's strange behavior.
He even thought, "I'm too ugly." The little lamb didn't
understand.*

*Finally, the little lamb fell asleep and had a dream.
In the dream, a beautiful angel appeared. "I know you
are confused, little lamb," said the angel. "You do not
understand your father's behavior. It is not because of
you. It's not good for children to be around adults
who drink poison water. Your father is sick. In order*

for him to be with you, he must stop drinking poison water." With those words, the angel sprinkled some beautiful magic sparkles over the little lamb and disappeared.

When Baby Lamb awoke, he felt much better. He was relieved to know, in his heart, he was not to blame for his father's behavior. With this new knowledge, he was once again able to play and eat his favorite foods. He was also able to sleep in his own bed. And, after a time, when his mother asked him if he wanted to visit his father again, the baby replied, "Only if Daddy behaves." Baby Lamb knew that children can be young and smart at the same time.

Why Storytelling Is Helpful

Metaphorical storytelling is an effective way to address traumatic memories and their responses and to teach problem solving. It also emphasizes resiliency strengths in children. As children listen to the stories, they have an opportunity to resonate with the problem–solving, empowered hero or heroine within themselves.

Storytelling also bypasses resistance by speaking to, as well as offering solutions to, overcoming a trauma without directly discussing *the* trauma. Additionally, stories convey hopeful messages, create positive physical changes within the body, and relax the listener. And, while the story illustrated above was written for a child, an adolescent is also receptive to its message.[1]

Stories also transform PTSD symptoms. For example, five-year–old Mark began to soil his pants after he had been molested by an older boy. He listened every night to his storytelling tape, and his symptoms surprisingly disappeared after one week. While this is an exceptional example of the positive effects of storytelling, clients usually experience some level of relief after hearing their stories.

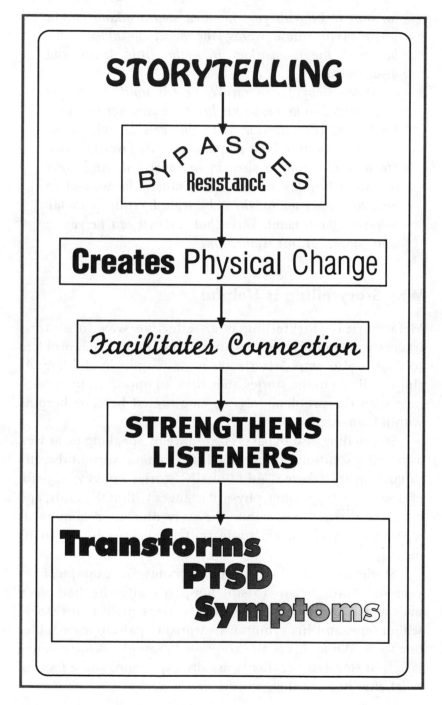

STORYTELLING

BYPASSES Resistance

Creates Physical Change

Facilitates Connection

STRENGTHENS LISTENERS

Transforms PTSD Symptoms

Stories can be taped for later listening, shared personally, or utilized in a group setting. And children can also create their own stories, enlightening themselves as well as their helpers.

How to Create a Metaphorical Story

Gathering Information

Before formulating a metaphorical story, gather background information. For example, Misty, age seven, has been living in foster care for six months. She complains of stomach pain and has been overheard crying in her sleep. Misty also reports nightmares and is visibly shaken when they occur. On the next page is a list of sample background questions answered by Misty and other sources. Later, this information will be symbolically communicated throughout her metaphorical story.

With this information, a therapeutic story can be written which resonates with Misty's unconscious. A story includes 11 necessary elements.

(1) The story describes the child's PTSD symptoms.

For example, Misty's nightmares were terrifying and disruptive. She often complained of a stomach ache and became emotional when she was lightly bruised or cut.

In Misty's story, the heroine would exhibit similar problems. While the main character (heroine) may be nonhuman, it would have nightmares, experience stomach aches, and excessively worry over small ailments.

(2) The child identifies with an inviting and lovable main character (hero or heroine).

The child's idea of a heroine is worked into the story. For example, Misty would be drawn to a story where her favorite doll is the story's central figure.

Without overemphasizing conventional stereotypes, many times boys respond to stories where the main characters are firefighters, policemen, or other hero

Sample Questions and Answers

Background Questions About the Child	Answers from Misty or Others
The presenting problem is:	physical abuse by mother
The presenting symptoms are:	nightmares, somatic complaints
The family situation is:	father in prison, mother absent, child and siblings live in foster care, maternal grandmother had been primary caregiver in past, but is now unable to care for Misty
Life before abuse:	many moves, lived with grandmother longer than with anyone else, happier at grandmother's
Likes and dislikes are:	*Likes:* kittens, puppies, hamburgers, watching TV, mother and grandmother *Dislikes:* scary programs, liver, leaving mother
Favorite activities are:	playing Barbie with friends, birthday parties, picking strawberries and flowers, watching cartoons

archetypes, who work through their problems because they think fast or use physical strength. Girls, on the other hand, generally enjoy problem-solving heroines, such as wise princesses or powerful unicorns, who are smart and kind but assertive and clever.

(3) A symbol which embodies the incident or person who caused the child to be hurt.

In the story *Baby Lamb and His Father*, the angry ram symbolizes the alcoholic father who hurt Ryan. Misty's physical abuse could be described in her story as an angry hurricane or an out-of-control vehicle. There are several ways to describe the child's pain or her abuser, and part of the task of writing a meaningful story for a child is knowing the child.

(4) The story is consistent with the child's problem.

Misty's problem is that she acquired maladaptive posttrauma stress responses as a result of her trauma. Misty's *goal* is to know she is safe now, while understanding at a deep level that she was never responsible for her mother's behavior. Misty's story would include an experience which frightened the heroine. The story would further describe how the character developed problems and later overcame them, due to her insight, intelligence, and quick thinking.

(5) The heroine is described as the same gender as child.

Since Misty is female, the main character of her story is female. The name of the main character, or heroine, would be a name that Misty liked, such as Barbie, mentioned earlier. For very young children, the main character may even have the same name.

(6) The story has an emphasis on resilience characteristics.

Misty is very resilient; she is kind and helpful. She

has already developed some interests that serve her well. These strengths can be used to describe the main character and to emphasize how problems are resolved.

(7) The use of settings is consistent with child's idea of safety and security.

The countryside and flowers are positive images for Misty. Later this positive imagery can be used to help her relax. Misty's story will reflect a place where the main character can feel secure. The safe setting can also be described in the story as a place where she can solve her problems.

(8) The story outlines a plan to overcome the problem.

Within the story, the heroine will be able to become aware of or understand how to rethink or reframe her problem. The story will describe how she learned that she was not to blame, or how she came to understand that she had the knowledge within herself to overcome her fears. There are thousands of ways in which overcoming a problem can be described.

A metaphorical story is consistent with how the child might solve a problem. For example, Misty would not resonate with a story that included resolving a problem through force. Rather, she would relate to a woodland animal with magical dust or drinks.

(9) The story emphasizes the child's mastery of the problem.

Positive resolutions created through mastering the problem are emphasized. For example, the heroine is rewarded in some manner, recognizes her own strengths, or copes with her problems more positively.

(10) The story contains a messenger who conveys the solution to the child's problem.

Since Misty related that she felt warmly toward her grandmother, the message bearer within her metaphorical story might be a kindly owl, or a fairy godmother. Message bearers can be described in metaphorical stories as changes in nature or inanimate objects, such as a flying carpet or talking umbrella. If the child identifies with the messenger, she will hear the message.

(11) Cultural appropriateness is maintained.

If Misty is American Indian, descriptive words and familiar nouns are used within the story. For example, Misty's message bearer could be an "ancestor." Include a culturally appropriate ritual when possible, as well as the name of songs or games the main character would sing or play.

Writing Your Own Story

A powerful way to understand the strengths of metaphorical storytelling, is to write a metaphorical story yourself. Writing your own story can bring about very positive recognitions.

For example, one woman in a training workshop shared that she became aware of her resistance to making changes in her life after writing her story. Another workshop participant described getting in touch with an unresolved loss. Someone else described his renewed confidence after identifying his resiliency strengths. Writing a personal story can be very enlightening.

When you write your own story, include the elements described earlier in the chapter, remembering to emphasize the heroine's (hero's) mastery over the problem. On page 68 is a list of elements you should include as you write your story. After completing the story, notice what you experienced emotionally and physically. You may wish to tape the story.

How to Impart a Story

Good timing is essential when sharing a metaphorical story. Stories that sound contrived can be sensed and dismissed in short order by a child or adolescent. Keep in mind, imparting

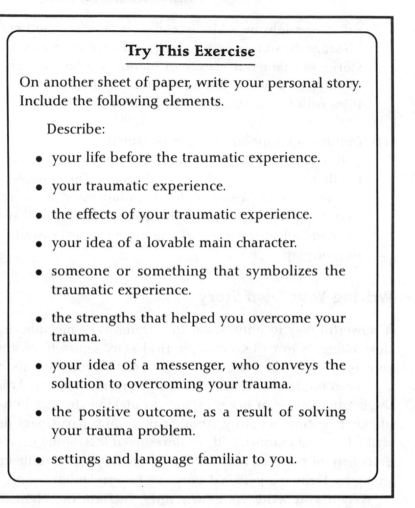

Try This Exercise

On another sheet of paper, write your personal story. Include the following elements.

Describe:

- your life before the traumatic experience.

- your traumatic experience.

- the effects of your traumatic experience.

- your idea of a lovable main character.

- someone or something that symbolizes the traumatic experience.

- the strengths that helped you overcome your trauma.

- your idea of a messenger, who conveys the solution to overcoming your trauma.

- the positive outcome, as a result of solving your trauma problem.

- settings and language familiar to you.

the story will not be effective if the child is not in a safe setting, or is otherwise distracted. If a child reports she was unable to understand the story, rewrite the story in order to make it clearer. Stories are helpful to share at the end of counseling sessions, in order to emphasize a point made during the hour, and at other times when two people are engaged in a routine activity.

⮜ • *Mike* • ⮞

Richard shared a story with Mike, age 15, as they traveled to court one day. Mike was visiting the judge

because he had been arrested for buying marijuana.
Richard, his residential counselor, thinking a metaphori-
cal story might assist Mike in becoming more aware
of his recent behavior, shared a story about a favorite
uncle.

Richard's uncle, a farmer, had learned not to
antagonize the bulls on the farm after a rather harrowing
experience. Within the story was the message, that taking
unnecessary chances can lead to bigger problems. Richard
related later to colleagues, that while he wasn't sure
if the young man resonated with the story, it was curious
that Mike seemed to stop buying marijuana.

Caregivers can develop stories to be heard at specific
moments, such as bedtime, when a child feels more nervous,
or when she will be facing a particular challenge. Stories can
also diffuse a child's agitated state. Taping stories gives children something to hear when the helper is not present. Taped
stories are accessible. One adolescent recently asked her counselor to make her another tape to replace the one that had
been worn out.

Storytelling Resonates with Symbolism

Metaphorical storytelling draws upon associations to everyday
symbols. Symbolic associations are similar to the way dream-
ing creates mental pictures during sleep. Pictures or movies
within dreams are simply symbols given personal meaning in
order to problem solve. Metaphorical stories are different
because they are consciously created to help children.

Metaphorical storytelling, responsibly formulated and
imparted, actually bypasses resistance and fosters healing in
traumatized children. It is an indispensable tool when helping
young people. An Audiotape Checklist is provided on the following pages to assist in the taping of stories.

Audiotape Checklist

(1) The child is prepared to listen to the stories.

An invitation is extended, especially to older children and adolescents. For example, "I invite you to find a comfortable place to rest. It may be in your room, or outside on the grass. Notice that as you become comfortable, your body relaxes into the grass, sofa, chair, etc.... Take a couple deep breathes and exhale any stress, worries." The helper can elaborate before proceeding into the story. (The listener is reassured that she is *not* being hypnotized. This can also be done when she is given the tape.)

(2) The helper lets the child know she can share the tape with anyone.
It is her choice. (This may be said directly on the tape or written down in a note to the child when she receives the tape.)

(3) The helper lets her know she can turn off the tape at any time.
(Included with the information in number 2.)

(4) It is not important if the child pays rigid attention to the story.
(Again, included with information in numbers 2 and 3.)

(5) The helper eases the child into the story.

The helper should acclimate the child so that she is relaxed and comfortable. This can be done can by saying, "Very good. I'd like to begin by telling you the name of the first story on this side of the tape," or "Many times I begin my story by just saying, 'Now, there once lived a young lady,' etc...."

(6) Adolescents need to be strongly cautioned not to drive or operate equipment while listening to the tape.

Story listening is often a very relaxing experience.

(7) Several stories can be imparted on the tape.

Helpers should keep in mind distractibility based on developmental stages. For example, a 10 or 15 minute tape is adequate for a young child, while adolescents can listen to 30 minutes of stories quite easily.

(8) The helper needs to sound as though she is enjoying sharing the story and to personalize the tape by directly addressing the listener.

Children like to hear words of encouragement; the helper should not be afraid to drop in remarks such as, "Good," "Great," or "You're on your way."

Notes

1.   N. Davis, *Once upon a time…Therapuetic stories to heal abused children* (Oxon Hill, MD: Author, 1988).

Overcoming Adversity through Resiliency

We know that children with proper support can thrive in spite of being traumatized. Many children who have faced adversity not only move beyond their trauma but seem to become stronger individuals. This ability to thrive in the face of adversity, to overcome a traumatic childhood, is called *resilience*.

Bonnie Bernard, in her publication *Fostering Resiliency in Kids: Protective Factors in the Family, School, and Community*, identifies a number of attributes of resilient children, including responsiveness, flexibility, empathy and caring, communication skills, and a sense of humor. *Resilience*—ultimately, is the ability to face life with a will to win, to see life's obstacles as challenges, and to be able to bounce back from setbacks.[1]

We have all known resilient children. They have an air of invulnerability and an indomitable will to survive. They seem to attract adults to them with their humor and congeniality. Their competence and intelligence are unmistakable. They are resourceful and they seem to find ways to overcome or use stress to their advantage.

Rosa

Rosa is a resilient child. Her history includes physical and emotional abuse. Her father, a chronic alcoholic who had sexually abused her, left the family when she was eight years old. Her mother, overwhelmed with the responsibility

73

Parentified

of caring for her children, often left Rosa, age 12, in charge of her four small siblings for weeks at a time.

During one of her mother's long absences, the child welfare workers discovered Rosa caring for her siblings alone. The children were placed in out-of-home care.

Rosa was unable to acclimate to a foster home and was sent to a group home. She was popular with the staff and the children and did well in school. She was a self-directed child who showed initiative. She was generally able to use the support of adults to her advantage. Her sense of humor also endeared her to housemates.

She was angry at being separated from her siblings, however, and resentful of the house rules that made her "feel like a child." She would often complain, "I've been taking care of myself and my brothers and sisters since I can remember. I washed their clothes, fed them, and stayed up with them when they were sick. You people are just like that foster mother. You are trying to turn me into a child. I've been an adult for a long time."

Rosa had never assumed the role of a child. She needed help to move toward an age appropriate status. Her role as surrogate mother to her siblings, while difficult, had allowed her to feel good about herself. It had given her self-esteem.

The task of her caregivers was to find a way to help Rosa use her determination and resourcefulness to her own advantage. Her goal was to learn that she could behave like a 12-year-old and still maintain her sense of mastery over the world.

Trauma Is Only Part of the Story

Promote Resilience

There are many variables that promote resilience and protect children from the impact of childhood trauma. Some of these are a nurturing and caring environment; the presence of role models; access to resources; effectiveness in work, play, and relationships; and having an opportunity to contribute and be seen by others as a worthy person. Others include healthy expectations and a positive outlook, self-esteem, an internal locus of control, and problem–solving skills.

One important protective factor is the quality of care a child receives after a traumatic experience. There are many resilient children, like Rosa, who can realize that, in spite of their trauma, they can acquire new skills. Many times, these skills emerge as a result of their experience. The following are examples of these resilient characteristics.

Humor and Social Competence   (1)

Resilient children are more adaptable than other children and are more likely to establish positive relationships with caring adults. Resilient children know how to recruit helpers. One way they accomplish this is through humor.[2]

Humor is an important tool. It allows a child to deflect pain by making fun of it; thereby taking some control. Humor also attracts others; everyone likes a funny person. Children who can engage adults are more likely to receive positive feedback, which in turn enhances their sense of *social competence*. Children can also use humor inappropriately. It is important for care-givers to teach them when to use humor in a positive way.

The Ability to Plan and Problem-Solving Skills   (2)

Young women who take on domestic responsibilities, includ-ing care for younger siblings, feel a sense of self–worth and a feeling of competence. Age appropriate responsibility gives children the opportunity to develop self–esteem while learning *planning skills*. Researcher Michael Rutter [1984] found that chil-dren who can plan for the future have a better chance of being successful later in life. He found that "especially in the popula-tion of abused and neglected girls who later became healthy adults, the presence of planning skills resulted in their plan-ning marriages to nondeviant men."[3]

Children who care for younger siblings, like Rosa, have to be able to solve problems. *Problem-solving skills* are needed in order to survive on the streets. How often have you marveled at the fast thinking of children who have survived their crime ridden and violent environments? It is important for caregivers to help children translate their street smarts to pro-social problem-solving and planning. Often traumatized children do not have role models for healthy problem solving. This is something they must find from other caring adults.

Werner and Smith [1982] in their book, *Overcoming the Odds: High Risk Children from Birth to Adulthood*, state that self-esteem and self-efficacy grew when children were given responsible positions commensurate with abilities. This was true, whether it was part-time paid work or managing the household. Giving children duties to do in the home or cottage is an important part of helping children to develop problem-solving skills. This can include life planning projects, playing games that involve the ability to sort through options, and other activities that support the development of analytical thinking.[4]

Adaptive Distancing

Adaptive distancing is a strategy used by children to distance themselves from their family dysfunction. Beardslee and Podorefsky [1988] found that resilient children "were able to distinguish clearly between themselves and their own experiences, and their parents illness."[5]

Most children have an extremely difficult time separating themselves from their biological roots. Resilient children appear to have a good sense of their personal identity, which helps them through the separation process. Adaptive distancing is more of a relief than an additional trauma for resilient children. They can and do see themselves as separate from their parents' problems and/or illness, and realize they did not cause nor can they cure them.

Distancing expresses itself in many ways. Often, children from dysfunctional homes will acquire adoption fantasies, unconsciously choosing not to identify with their family's pathology. Distancing may also include refusing to go home for visits or not answering phone calls from parents. Later the decision to go to another state for college or join the armed forces may be a way to gain distance from an actively dysfunctional family. Many adult children of trauma simply move far away from their parents as soon as they are able. They maintain a physical, as well as psychological, distance.

It is important for caregivers to support a sense of autonomy with children who are not able to psychologically distance themselves from their family. This may be accomplished by simply reinforcing that they did not cause their family's problems, they cannot cure these problems, and their lives can be different from the lives led by their parents.

It is also important for caregivers to support the notion that loving one's parents does not mean being like them in every way. A child should be given the opportunity to express herself about her parents' negative traits if it helps the child create a sense of independence from the family. It is even more helpful to reinforce this independence when a child's stress reactions are triggered on home visits.

Many traumatized children are conflicted about loving their family and hating their family's behaviors. The child care professional, however, must "walk a thin line" between reinforcing the child's adaptive distancing and continuing to support the child's love for her biological family.

An Inner Locus of Control

(4)

Children growing up in chaotic homes are often given mixed messages. For example, they are told that things are all right after Dad has just beaten up Mom. Or they are informed that nothing happened when Brother came home drunk and wrecked the car. They know instinctively that in these circumstances adults may not be telling the truth. But because they are children, they disregard their own perceptions.

These children grow up not trusting their own perceptions. They look to others to tell them what to think. After years of being told that their sense of reality is wrong, they no longer can think on their own without help. The obvious is no longer obvious to them. These children are called *outer directed*; they do not trust their own perceptions about life.

Some of these children do not believe they can change their circumstances; instead, they feel like victims of their situation. Their hopelessness leads them to acquire a passive stance in life. These children can grow up to marry abusive spouses and accept their spouse's view of reality.

Resilient children learn to trust their own perceptions in the face of their family's denial. They are able to separate from the family dysfunction. These children are said to have an inner locus of control. What they do, and how they think, is dictated by their internal signals and not by what others tell them. They are unlikely to marry abusive spouses.

An inner locus of control means maintaining a sense of self in the midst of chaos and denial. It is important for traumatized children to develop the ability to see a reality separate from the one that their family has told them to believe. For example, when substance abuse is involved, the whole family may be denying their dysfunction. Caregivers need to reinforce a sense of personal reality for traumatized children.

Spirituality

Spirituality is important for any child but especially for traumatized children. We know that many children who were traumatized and later became successful adults had a deep and abiding belief in God. Resilient individuals use their faith to maintain a positive vision of a meaningful life and to successfully negotiate an abundance of emotionally hazardous experiences.

Spirituality and involvement with religious organizations is a way children find much needed meaning and security. The belief in God gives children the sense that at least one entity is 100% on their side. God is the only supportive parent many traumatized children have been able to rely on.[6]

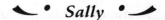

～• Sally •～

Sally is an adult child of abusive alcoholic parents. Additionally, her family was involved with criminal behavior; often selling stolen goods. She reflected, "If it hadn't been for my belief in God, I wouldn't have survived my childhood. You can't imagine what that house was like. The cursing and hitting were constant. There were no rules to live by. But when I prayed to God, I could escape my family and find some meaning for the suffering we all went through. When I went to church, I discovered a new and healthy family. In fact, I found a number of families to join. My church also allowed me to meet older women who could be role models; something I didn't have at home."

For children like Sally, a loving God gives them a way to reframe their pain. It gives their suffering meaning and assists in their healing process.

High Expectations and a Sense of a Future

Caregivers know the value of *high expectations* and a positive outlook on life. Helping children who were traumatized to notice the best in themselves, and to realize their possibilities, is extremely important.

Traumatized children often come from families where they received negative feedback. Children grow up hearing they "won't amount to anything," and "not to expect much from life." When someone stands up for one of these children, it makes a big difference.

◣ • *Linda* • ◢

Linda, an incest survivor, states why she feels successful. "My mother is an alcoholic. She abused all of us and totally intimidated my father. She said I'd end up as a prostitute. She made fun of my efforts to do well in school, telling me I was wasting my time.

"If it hadn't been for my grandmother, my mother would have been right. Grandma lived close by and I

spent every free moment with her. She told me stories about the successful people in our family. Grandma also taught me to believe that I had a bright future before me, in spite of what my parents said. She said that I could do anything I wanted with my life and that I needed to follow my dreams. We used to sit on the roof of her building and she would say, 'Honey, there's nothing bigger than you and those stars. Nothing that can come between you and your dreams, if you believe in yourself!'

"*My grandmother died before I graduated from medical school, but she's with me every day of my life. She is the voice of love and affirmation which helped me build a ladder out of that terrible, angry, and despairing family.*"

Linda's grandmother gave her a sense of her own possibilities. Traumatized children need support in their lives. Parents who abuse their children are not likely to encourage them. A caregiver must be that "voice of possibility" for children. One of the most powerful roles a caregiver can play, is to be the messenger who expresses those high expectations and helps a child reach for the stars.

A Significant Caring Adult

In the book *Overcoming the Odds: High Risk Children from Birth to Adulthood*, Werner and Smith [1992] state that the resilient youngsters in their study "all had at least one person in their lives who accepted them unconditionally, regardless of temperamental idiosyncrasies, physical attractiveness, or intelligence."[7]

The presence of a *significant caring adult* in the life of traumatized children is perhaps *the* one most important support for resilient children. Successful resilient children find parent surrogates to help raise them. For some it can be an aunt or grandparent, but for others it can be a teacher, coach, minister, neighbor, or counselor. It does not matter who it is, as long as someone is there to help the children negotiate the travails of life with wisdom and compassion, and the children know that the person is 100% on their side.

❧ • *Henry* • ❧

A successful contractor, Henry grew up with a physically abusive father. His coach was his voice of affirmation. "Coach Menendez put me here today. My father used to beat my mother and me all the time. We never knew when he was going to explode. All of a sudden he would erupt. Even now, when I hear loud voices, I tense as though he is still around.

"My father told me I was nothing but a bum and I'd never amount to anything. I believed him and lived up to his low expectation of me. When I met Coach, I was an angry, violent, 13-year-old, who was barely passing his courses and clearly on his way to serious trouble. Coach helped me turn that anger to positive use on the football field. When my father told me I was useless, Coach helped me to see that my father was way beyond insecure, and that it was not the way I needed to see myself. He taught me how to protect myself from the negativity within my family.

"Basically, Coach became the father I didn't have. When I had problems, I went to him, not to my father or mother. He helped me when I had girl problems, difficulties with my teachers, and he persuaded me to see a therapist when my PTSD symptoms threatened to overwhelm me."

Henry's coach reframed his life circumstance, so he was able to learn how to live in his family without becoming like his family. He taught Henry how to see his father as an alcoholic with a disease, and that Henry did not have to be like his father. Helping children reframe their negative perceptions about themselves and life is essential to recovery.

Every caregiver can make a difference by being a significant caring adult for children. Supporting the development of resiliencies in children will help them in their recovery and launch them on the way to successful lives. The checklist on the next pages may be helpful to you.

Resiliency Building Checklist

Emphasizing resilience traits reinforces positive coping skills and self-esteem. These are some suggestions:

- The child is assigned small tasks appropriate to her skills and interests.

- The helper notices and remarks favorably on the child's appropriate humor.

- The helper provides at least two solutions to a problem and allows the child to choose one.

- The child is asked to provide at least two solutions to a problem.

- The helper introduces hypothetical planning exercises.

- New concepts about how to live one's life are introduced. For example, the helper can take the child to museums, a college campus, ethnic communities, the library—letting her experience options.

- The helper introduces a hobby; teaching the child kite or doll making, knitting, wood-working, writing, ceramics, sewing.

- The child's perceptions of reality are affirmed when the helper asks her what she thinks and believes.

- The helper reinforces the child's skills by asking her to demonstrate, for example, how to throw a ball, sing, write a story, tell a joke, etc....

- The helper and child play board games. Games like "Monopoly," "Chutes and Ladders," and "Sorry" reinforce problem–solving skills.

- The helper can share stories about people who successfully overcame difficult experiences and adversity.

- The child needs to be provided with opportunities to express her spirituality. Some children may desire a private place where they can pray. Still others want to be taken to church. A child may also need to share her spirituality with another person.

- All accomplishments, large or small, can be celebrated.

- The helper can send a "thinking of you card" to the child.

Notes

Resiliency
References

1. B. Bernard, *Fostering resiliency in kids: Protective factors in the family, school, and community* (Portland, OR: Northwest Regional Educational Laboratory, 1991).

2. *Ibid.*

3. E. Werner, & R. Smith, *Overcoming the odds: High risk children from birth to adulthood* (New York: Cornell University Press, 1992). M. Rutter, "Resilient children," *Psychology Today* (March 1984), 57–65, as cited in B. Bernard, *Fostering resiliency in kids: Protective factors in the family, school, and community* (Portland, OR: Northwest Regional Educational Laboratory, 1991).

4. E. Werner, & R. Smith, *Overcoming the odds: High risk children from birth to adulthood* (New York: Cornell University Press, 1992).

5. W. Beardslee, & D. Podorefsky, "Resilient adolescents whose parents have serious affective and other psychiatric disorders: Importance of self-nurturing and relationships," *American Journal of Psychiatry, 145*(1) (1988), 63–69.

6. E. Werner, & R. Smith, *Overcoming the odds: High risk children from birth to adulthood* (New York: Cornell University Press, 1992).

7. *Ibid.*

∼ • 8 • ∼

Dealing with Past Trauma
as Adult Caregivers

> *We have learned to place in the foreground*
> *the personality of the doctor himself as*
> *the curative or harmful factor. What is*
> *now demanded is his own transformation, the*
> *self-education of the educator.*
>
> — *C. G. Jung[1]*

Advocating in behalf of children is complex work. While a career helping children has its rewards, it can also be emotionally draining. Altruistic intentions are often behind choosing this profession. Statements, such as "wanting to make a difference," or "helping the world become a better place for kids," are frequently written on child advocacy job applications. These days, however, child care professionals are confronted by problems more severe than those of their colleagues who worked 25 years ago. One social worker, Maria Iriarte, LCSW, who formerly worked at the Roxey Bolton Rape Treatment Center, at Jackson Memorial Hospital in Miami, Florida, shares concerns about the increasing severity of her clients' presenting problems.

For example, she has counseled greater numbers of younger children who are impregnated by their family members. Some of the pregnant girls are 10 years old and far along in their pregnancies before they receive any counseling assistance. Most of these children have already experienced multiple traumas.

Current child welfare conditions require professionals to be streetwise and book–smart, as well as positive thinkers, in the face of adversity. Caregivers traumatized as children will often bring a positive attitude to their work, in addition to their own understanding about trauma recovery. Helpers who have taken time to examine their past have a special wisdom that allows them to intervene carefully with traumatized young people. Conversely, they need to be alert to the "on–the–job" liabilities their past brings to their work.

Most child advocates sincerely want to help children. Embracing good intentions is positive, and while it is helpful to bring these qualities to the job, there are other considerations which have as much impact on children, such as the childhood experiences of the child care advocate.

Self-Education of the Educator

Because of their histories, child advocates can be great spokespersons for the rights of children, yet they can overlook the road blocks created by these same histories. Caregivers who have been traumatized in childhood usually have the best intentions when they enter the child advocacy field. They are often unaware that their former trauma(s) can impact their job performance. Here are some examples caused by fallout from childhood trauma.

Don Quixote Syndrome

Formerly traumatized individuals may acquire a heightened sense of justice. This awareness may translate to a *Don Quixote* approach to work, which is exhausting for the workers and coworkers. Magical thinking about one's abilities to help sets the stage for a person to feel used and tired. It is not helpful to have unrealistic expectations about changing the world.[2]

⟍• *Annette* •⟋

Annette, a 48-year-old child welfare supervisor, paid a price for her hypervigilant advocacy when she first became a social worker. "Because I'd been left in the dark about my own placement in an orphanage when I was six, I felt compelled to work on changing the child welfare system, immediately. I was concerned that children should not fall through the cracks, as I had. I wanted to spare all children my pain.

"I worked 70 hours a week and straight into an ulcer. But I thought everyone worked that hard. It seemed natural. Over time, my exhausting work schedule took a toll on me, physically and emotionally. I learned about pacing myself the hard way. Now I understand that a well utilized 40-hour work week is more effective than an exhausting 70 hours; which, after a while, leads to mistakes."

Traumatized children often tolerate higher levels of stress in order to sustain themselves during their childhood. As adults they become confused when other people do not operate under the same pressure. Working regular hours, removing "struggle" from their lives, becoming aware of early stress signals, and understanding personal limitations are four important recovery goals for helpers.

Separatism

Recovery from Posttraumatic Stress Disorder is a meaningful accomplishment. However, it should not separate coworkers. Feeling special because of one's past condition is a sign that a trauma survivor has missed something in her recovery process. This perspective stops people from working together as a team and diminishes the work of those who did not have the misfortune to be traumatized as children. It also creates a "we against them" perspective which does not help the most important people—the children.

～ • *Cindy* • ～

Cindy states, "I was one of the founding members of my adult survivor of incest support group. I began my recovery work in the mid-80s and felt a lot of anger about my abuse. I kind of fell into an AA, 12-step approach to my recovery, and over time noticed that I ignored friendships with people who had not been molested in childhood. They weren't in my group. Because of my anger, I know I was a turnoff at staff meetings and, frankly, I didn't want to hear what nonsurvivors had to recommend about their clients. I felt that I was the expert. In retrospect, I know I was pretty obnoxious."

Oppositional Behavior

Often, people who have been traumatized as children are angry. Anger is a natural outgrowth of abuse, but it needs to be dealt with because it can be projected on the job. For example, some adult survivors may resist supervision because their boss is an authority figure. Or they may have disputes with clients who remind them of someone in their past. Bridges are often burned when anger is expressed inappropriately in court or on a home visit. *Oppositional behavior* needs to be examined and modified, so that valuable time is not wasted when advocating in behalf of children.

Inability to Show Empathy

Scott W. Allen, Ph.D., a staff psychologist with the Metro–Dade Police Department in Miami, Florida, counsels adults with PTSD. Dr. Allen comments that sometimes law enforcement professionals who were traumatized as children have *difficulty being empathetic.*

Intolerance is most apparent in individuals who may do a cursory intervention with a traumatized child because they have difficulty tolerating someone else's pain. They will deflect their feelings by making a cynical remark or spending as little time as possible on a case. Some advocates have gone so far as to blame the child victim for her trauma. An example includes a tiny group of rape counselors who remark that adolescent prostitutes "are asking to be raped."

Inappropriate Discipline.

(5)

Individuals traumatized as children may use *inappropriate methods of discipline* because they cannot completely transform early impressions they received from their own caregivers. For example, one child care supervisor was appalled to learn that his house parent, thinking it was a perfectly appropriate act, locked a child in a closet. When questioned, the house parent remarked that he believed it was one of the better things he learned from his parents, who had physically abused him during childhood. This house parent was able to understand the inappropriateness of overt physical punishment. It took him a while longer to understand that locking a child in a closet was also a form of child abuse.

Compulsive Caregiving

(6)

There is an old adage about the doctor who overlooks his own care because he is busy treating everyone else. This can also apply to advocates traumatized as children, when attempting to heal their pain by helping others. Unfortunately, this round-about way of dealing with personal hurt is not helpful.

Work can be their avoidance behavior. "Too many children need my help," or "I've just got to see this kid today," are statements that validate the reasons for working late or on weekends.

Ignoring personal care can prevent someone from resolving a marital conflict, or simply taking a vacation. Scheduling time to include a well-rounded life experience takes practice for many professionals traumatized as children.

Additionally, we have all known advocates who will neglect their physical health, and/or avoid changing her social status, because they are more willing to suffer through work than tackle the effects of their childhood trauma. Being around people who would rather work than face their problems can be irritating for coworkers who are spending time with their children or taking "mental health" days. But more importantly, it does not enhance the life of the individual who practices this behavior.

Hypervigilance and Perfectionism

People who were traumatized in childhood often feel that they should be perfect. This may be a result of being severely punished for making mistakes or simply as a compensation for growing up in very "imperfect" homes. These people will scan their environment continually for cues that they have done something wrong. This fear will often cause them to become rigid in their thinking and fearful of other people. They may interpret comments made by supervisors, which are meant to be helpful, as criticism.

They may reject the opinions of their colleagues and fail to listen to the needs expressed by their clients because they do not want to appear "wrong" by taking corrective action, even when it is necessary. *Hypervigilance* and *perfectionism* are characteristics that need to be examined by professionals who were traumatized as children. The challenge for these professionals is to become flexible and forgiving of themselves.

Emotional and Physical Boundary Crossing

Child advocacy work includes managing crisis. Crisis intervention can be exhausting and confusing, especially when clients are confused, delusional, agitated, and/or impulsive. This can set up the adult advocate to become a "rescuer." Unfortunately, she can often feel "persecuted" by her clients as well.

One of the goals in recovering from childhood trauma is to understand and practice maintaining clear *emotional and physical boundaries.* Child care professionals must pay special attention to not crossing these lines by overidentifying with clients or their family members. Otherwise they can feel victimized or even persecuted by the same people they are trying to help.

Foster parents who were traumatized as children are at high risk of crossing these boundaries because, as surrogate parents, they are asked to maintain an emotional decorum while caring for a child 24 hours a day. An overidentification with a foster child can occur if a foster parent has not resolved her early issues of abandonment, which may have accompanied her childhood trauma. Foster parent training and support along these lines would help to minimize the pain associated with the eventual separation from a child.

Doubting Professional Judgment

A tendency to *doubt professional judgment* is common among formerly traumatized individuals. Confidence does not come easily to an adult who suffered catastrophic loss or trauma. In spite of the fact that a child advocate may be correct in her judgment, she may back down unnecessarily when challenged by someone who appears more self–assured. Or she will defer to someone less qualified but more confident to speak, for example, in court.

Some parents of traumatized children are able to continue a reign of terror because they are charmingly sociopathic. It takes an individual with strong convictions to confront these people. Professionals must be able to trust their judgment under pressure.

Denial

Caregivers who were traumatized in childhood need to be cautious about denying the impact of their earlier trauma. Surprisingly, few human service professionals, ranging from psychiatrists to front line advocates, take advantage of ongoing therapy to enhance their work. In the case of caregivers traumatized as children, therapy is essential and will ultimately enhance their personal and professional life.

Many survivors of childhood trauma are in *denial* about the effects of their past terrifying experiences. Alcoholism, workaholism, and sex addictions are common among helping professionals when they deny they were effected by their childhood traumas.

It is truly helpful for previously traumatized professionals to participate in insight-oriented activities in order to understand how they, as professionals, can be most effective. Activities may include individual or group therapies. An insight-oriented exercise may mean periodic participation in self-awareness workshops. Or it may be a professional support group that generates self-examination.

"I worked in the child advocacy field for 10 years before I'd remembered my childhood abuse. In retrospect, I wonder how I managed the pressures at work and at home. I guess I didn't because I became aware of my trauma after I'd been suspended from my job. Therapy would have helped me all along, but I thought I'd finished myself when I finished graduate school." This remark was made by a child advocate who is taking time away from her career in order to reexamine her life.

Magical Thinking

A natural outgrowth from a childhood trauma is magical thinking. *Magical thinking* creates hope in a child whose immediate circumstances appear hopeless. It includes excessive fantasizing about her life in the future. Consequently, people can grow to adulthood and continue to believe that situations will improve rather magically.

One form of magical thinking is when someone chooses to notice only positive qualities in others. When people perceive life this way, they are denying reality and reinforcing their avoidance tendencies. Denying reality is what keeps the child going but very often holds the adult back. For example, a battered wife believes her abusive spouse will change if he is given more time in the relationship, or a parent believes that love without limits creates a self-disciplined child.

Children are sometimes placed in physical jeopardy because child advocates hope that parents have changed. The truth is a parent may not have changed, but if the advocate wears rose-colored glasses, they allow her to see only the *potential* for change. Unfortunately, potential does not mean reality.

Several years ago, I was incredulous when I overheard a child welfare professional tell a couple who had disclosed their sexual molestation of their five daughters that they (the parents) did not need agency intervention. The colleague stated that all they really needed was divine intervention. By the time the parents were reinterviewed, they had recanted their disclosure.

Admiring others is normal but magical thinkers often take it a step farther and *idealize* people. Idealizing another person is ultimately disappointing because human beings are fallible. Traumatized caregivers who idealize others feel betrayed and angry if someone they have placed "on a pedestal" makes a mistake.[3]

Reality Check

If you are a caregiver who was traumatized in childhood, you may find the checklist on page 94 helpful. Answering "yes" to any of these statements may indicate that further self-examination will benefit you in your work.

Formerly Traumatized Caregivers Give Their Suffering Meaning

Traumatized children ask a basic question: why did this happen to me? Adults who were traumatized as children can help them answer this question as role models who have found ways to give their own suffering meaning. While no one would wish to reexperience trauma, helpers often remark that *because of their trauma*, they have acquired a larger capacity for helping children. In spite of the "on-the-job" liabilities, helpers traumatized as children can be superior caregivers.

There are several ways in which formerly traumatized caregivers give their suffering meaning. For example, they often

Reality Checklist

- I often work more than 50 hours a week.
- I often feel victimized by my clients.
- I go into work on my days off or when I am ill.
- I am often angry at work.
- I think about my childhood trauma regularly.
- I've never been in therapy for my childhood trauma.
- I never verbalize my feelings about my childhood trauma.
- I think I am better qualified to help children than other professionals who have not been traumatized.
- Lately, I've been sniping at my clients and coworkers.
- I have difficulty understanding how people can leave their work at the office.
- I often tell my troubles to my clients.
- I ignore my most difficult cases because they are basically hopeless.
- I do not like to take time with repeat juvenile offenders or chronic welfare recipients.
- Some children are begging to be hit.
- I think psychotherapy is for crazy people.
- My coworkers and supervisor do not understand me.
- I am not appreciated enough by my clients.
- There is good in everybody.
- My childhood trauma never affected me.

understand a child's experience from a deeper perspective. This perspective includes knowing how reassuring it can feel to be on the receiving end of someone's concern. True compassion places someone in another's shoes without judgment.

Additionally, personal experience is useful when offering hope to a child who is undergoing her own recovery process. Personal knowledge allows advocates to speak concisely about PTSD.

❧ • *Duncan* • ❧

Duncan, a cottage parent at a treatment center, states, "Not too many people seem to understand PTSD. I mean, they know the diagnosis. The psychiatrist and social worker here talk about it all the time. But I'm not sure if they've experienced it themselves. I have, and I know how quickly someone can 'go off.' And I understand how difficult it is live in the present. I feel a lot of empathy for a kid who gets freaked. I know all about wanting to run like hell or wanting to kick the crap out of someone when I became frightened."

Another resilient trait seen in caregivers who were traumatized in childhood is *courage*. It takes courage not only to overcome trauma, but courage is needed when placing oneself in the position of working with traumatized children. Forces that can surface old trauma issues are often present at court or during child abuse investigations.

Caregivers who were traumatized in childhood also have *good instincts*. Susan, a child protection worker, states, "I think that child advocates who experienced trauma as children often rely on their instincts. I know my survival in childhood depended on it. Other workers won't admit it publicly, but they use their instincts with their training when they work with children."

Open-mindedness is another resilient trait in formerly traumatized caregivers who understand that there may not be one clear path toward recovery. A psychologist interviewed for this book remarked, "I'm always surprised at the difference in children. Had I not experienced my own childhood trauma, I wouldn't appreciate their uniqueness. I use a variety of therapeutic interventions when I work with traumatized children."

4)   Finally, caregivers who were traumatized in childhood bring *perseverance* and *patience* to their work. Society, as a whole, does not understand the importance of perseverance in child advocacy work. But patience is a byword for advocates who felt misunderstood when they were going through their traumatic experiences. These caregivers offer hope to children and will continue to advocate in their behalf after others have "thrown in the towel."

Helping Children Is Complex Work

Caregivers who were traumatized in childhood understand that helping children is a complicated task. It is often difficult to place a child in safe surroundings. It can be more difficult to help a child feel secure within herself. Caregivers who were exposed to childhood trauma know there are many factors to consider and negotiate in order to assist a child in experiencing the latter. Helpers who deal with their own recovery are in a unique position to articulate the complexities of this work.

Notes

1. H. Read, M. Fordham, G. Adler, & W. Mcquire, (Eds.), *The collected works of C. G. Jung, Bollinger Series XX* (Princeton, NJ: Princeton University Press, 1979).

2. Don Quixote, a fictional character whose exploits were set during the Spanish Inquisition, zealously attempted to right injustices. His quest was often misunderstood and his idealism, at times, was counterproductive.

3. R. Sedgwick, *The wounded healer: Countertransference from a Jungian perspective* (New York: Routledge, 1994).

﹏ • *References* • ﹏

Chapter 1

Annin, P. (1995, May 1). It's a scary world. *Newsweek*. 24–53.

Canton, M. (1995, January 1). Dad shot mom, 6–year–old testifies. *Albuquerque Journal*, p. B1.

Green, B. L. (1988). *Trauma and its wake: The study and treatment of posttraumatic stress disorder*. New York: Brunner/Mazel.

Leinwand, D. (1996, June 3). Survey finds Florida kids are poorly. *Miami Herald*, p. 1B & 6B.

McCardy, K. & Daro, D. (1994). *Current trends in child abuse reporting and fatalities: The results of the 1993 Annual Fifty State Survey*. Chicago: National Committee for the Prevention of Child Abuse.

Rivera, C. (1995, April 26). Abuse, a leading cause of death for small children: Study finds. *Miami Herald*, p. 1A & 6A.

Chapter 2

Begler, S., & Brant, M. (1994, September 26). You must remember this. *Newsweek*, p. 68.

Braun, B. (1986). *Issues in the psychotherapy of multiple personality disorder*. New York: American Psychiatric Press, Inc. p. 7

Caddell, J. M., Fountain, D. L., Karuntzos, G. T., & Dennis, M. L. (1994). *Prognostic significance of childhood abuse for current treatment of methadone clinics: A preliminary analysis* (unpublished manuscript).

Cannon, W. B. (1945). *The way of an investigator: A scientist's research.* New York: W. W. Norton.

Cannon, W. B. (1939). *The wisdom of the body.* New York: W. W. Norton.

Goldston, D. B., Turnquist, D. C., & Knutson, J. F. (1989). Presenting problems of sexually abused girls receiving psychiatric services. *Journal of Abnormal Psychology, 98* (3), 314–317.

Green, B. L. (1993). Identifying survivors at risk: Trauma and stressors across events. In J. P. Wilson and B. Raphael (Eds.) *International handbook of traumatic stress syndromes.* (135–144). New York: Plenum Press.

Horowitz, M. J. (1983). *Image formation and psychotherapy.* New York: Jason Aronson.

Hussey, F., Singer, M., & Petchers, M. (1989). The relationship between sexual abuse and substance abuse among psychiatrically hospitalized adolescents. *Child Abuse and Neglect, 13* (3), 319–325.

Rutter, M. (1983). Stress, coping and development: Some issues and some questions. In N. Garmezy & M. Rutter (Eds.), *Stress, coping and development in children.* New York: McGraw-Hill.

Chapter 3

Brohl, K. (1991). *Pockets of craziness: Investigating suspected incest.* New York: Lexington Books–MacMillan International.

Brohl-Hagans, K., & Case, J. (1988). *When your child has been molested: A parents' guide to healing and recovery.* New York: Lexington Books–MacMillan International.

Chapter 4

Brohl, K. (1991). *Pockets of craziness: Investigating suspected incest.* New York: Lexington Books–MacMillan International.

Brohl-Hagans, K., & Case, J. (1988). *When your child has been molested: A parents' guide to healing and recovery.* New York: Lexington Books–MacMillan International.

Erikson, E. H. (1950). *Childhood and society.* New York: W. W. Norton.

Freud, S. A. (1943). *A general introduction to psychoanalysis.* New York: Doubleday.

Horowitz, M. J. (1971). Phase-oriented treated of stress response syndromes. *American Journal of Psychotherapy, 27,* 506–515

Janet, P. (1925). *Psychological Healing* (vol. 1). New York: MacMillan Inc.

Peterson, K.; Prout, M., & Schwartz, R. (1981). *Post-traumatic stress disorder: A clinician's guide.* New York: Plenum Press.

Chapter 5

Brohl, K. (1991). *Pockets of craziness: Investigating suspected incest.* New York: Lexington Books–MacMillan International.

Conly, J. (1994, July). *Training Curriculum.* Miami, FL: Author.

Elias, M. (1994, November 29). Eyeing New Treatment for Trauma. *USA Today*, p. 1.

Haley, J., (1983). *Uncommon therapy: The psychiatric techniques of Milton H. Erickson.* New York: Brunner/Mazel Publisher.

Stone, G. (1994, May 9). Magic Fingers. *New York Magazine*, pp. 33–37.

Chapter 6

Barker, P. (1985). *Using metaphors in psychotherapy.* New York: Brunner/Mazel, Inc.

Conly, J. (1994, July). *Training Curriculum.* Miami, FL: Author.

Dideo, J. (1983). *Interpreting children's drawings.* New York: Brunner/Mazel, Inc.

Ertes, C. P. (1992). *Women who run with the wolves: Myths and stories of the wild woman archetypes.* New York: Ballantine.

Rosen, E. (1982). *My voice will go with you: The teaching tales of Milton H. Erickson, M.D.* New York: W. W. Norton.

Rossi, E., & Ryan, M. (1985). *Life reframing in hypnosis* (vol. II). New York: Irvington.

Ucko, L. (1991). Whose afraid of the big bad wolf? *Social Worker Magazine*, 36(5) 14–16.

Chapter 7

Anthony, E. J. (Ed.). (1974). *The child in his family: Children at psychiatric risk* (vol. 3). New York: John Wiley and Sons, Inc. pp. 529–544.

Anthony, E. J., & Cohler, B. J. (Eds.). (1987). *The invulnerable child.* New York: Guilford.

Beardslee, W., & Podorefsky, D. (1988). Resilient adolescents whose parents have serious affective and other psychiatric disorders: Importance of self–understanding and relationships. *American Journal of Psychiatry, 145*(1), 63–69.

Bernard, B. (1991). *Fostering resiliency in kids: Protective factors in the family, school, and community.* Oregon: Northwest Regional Educational Laboratory.

Brown, G. W., & Harris, T. O. (1978). *Social origins of depression.* New York: Basic Books.

Brown, G. W., Harris, T. O., & Bifulco, A. (1986). Long term effects of early loss of parent. In M. Rutter, C. E. Izard, & P. B. Read (Eds.), *Depression in young people: Developmental and clinical perspectives* (pp. 251–296). New York: Guilford.

Clark, R. (1983). *Family life and school achievement: Why poor black children succeed or fail.* Chicago: University of Chicago Press.

Comer, J. P. (1988). *Maggie's American dream.* New York: New American Library.

Dugan, T., & Coles, R. (1989). *The child in our times: studies in the development of resiliency.* New York: Brunner/Mazel.

Garmezy, N. (1974). The study of competence in children at risk for severe psychopathology. In E. J. Anthony & C. Koupernik (Eds.), *The child in his family: Children at psychiatric risk. The International Yearbook.* (77–98). New York: John Wiley and Sons, Inc.

Garmezy, N., & Rutter, M. (1983). *Stress, coping and development in children.* New York: McGraw–Hill.

Ianni, F. A. J. (1989). *The search for structure.* New York: The Free Press.

Rutter, M. (1984, March). Resilient children. *Psychology Today,* pp. 57–65.

Werner, E., & Smith, R. (1989). *Vulnerable but invincible: A longitudinal study of resilient children and youth.* New York: Adams, Bannister, and Cox.

Werner, E., & Smith, R. (1992). *Overcoming the odds: High risk children from birth to adulthood.* New York: Cornell University Press.

Williams, T., & Kornblum, W. (1985). *Growing up poor.* Lexington, MA: D. C. Heath.

Wolin, S., & Wolin, S. (1993). *The resilient self.* New York: Villard Books.

Chapter 8

Bass, E., & Davis, L. (1988). *The courage to heal: A guide for women of child sexual abuse*. New York: Harper & Row.

Brohl, K. (1991). *Pockets of craziness: Investigating suspected incest*. New York: Lexington Books–MacMillan International.

Greist, J. H. (1984). *Depression and its treatment*. New York: Warner Books.

Frankl, V. E. (1984). *Man's search for meaning*. New York: Washington Square Press.

O'Gorman, P., & Diaz, P. (1988). *Twelve-steps to self-parenting*. Deerfield Beach, FL: Health Communications, Inc.

Sedgwick, R. (1994). *The wounded healer: Countertransference from a Jungian perspective*. New York: Routledge.

Whitfiled, C. L. (1985). *Healing the child within*. Deerfield Beach, FL: Health Communications, Inc.

∼• *Other Resources* •∼

Al-Anon Family Groups. (1994). *From survival to recovery: Growing up in an alcoholic home.* New York: Al-Anon World Service.

Anthony, E. J., & Cohler, B. J. (Eds.). (1987). *The invulnerable child.* New York: The Guilford Press.

Bettelheim, B. (1989). *The uses of enchantment: The meaning and importance of fairy tales.* New York: Random House, Inc.

Bradshaw, J. (1988). *Bradshaw on healing the shame that binds you.* Deerfield Beach, FL: Health Communications, Inc.

Cannon, W. (1932). *The wisdom of the body.* New York: W. W. Norton.

Child Welfare League of America. (1992). *Children at the front: A different view of the war on alcohol and drugs.* Washington, DC: Author.

Courtois, C. A. (1988). *Healing the incest wound: Adult survivors in therapy.* New York: W. W. Norton.

Dugan, T. & Coles, R. (1989). *The child in our times.* New York: Brunner/Mazel.

Finklehor, D. (1979). *Sexually victimized children.* New York: Free Press.

Forward, D., & Buck, C. (1979). *Betrayal of innocence: Incest and its devastation.* New York: Penguin Books.

MacFarlane, K., & Waterman, J. (1986). *Sexual abuse of young children.* New York: Guilford Press.

Rossi, E. L. (1986). *The psychobiology of mind-body healing: New concepts of therapeutic hypnosis.* New York: W. W. Norton.

Satir, V. (1976). *Conjoint family therapy: A guide to theory and technique.* Palo Alto, CA: Science and Behavior Book.

Sgroi, S. (1982). *Handbook of clinical intervention in child sexual abuse*. Lexington, MA: Lexington Books.

Van der Kolk, B. A. (1988). The biological response to trauma. In F. Ochberg (Ed.), *Post-traumatic therapy and victim violence*. New York: Brunner/Mazel.

Wolin, S., & Wolin, S. (1993). *The resilient self: How survivors of troubled families rise above adversity*. New York: Villard Press.

◡ • *About the Author* • ◡

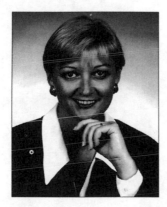

Kathryn Brohl, M.A., is a licensed Marriage and Family Therapist practicing in Miami, Florida. She has authored or coau-
thored, *Pockets of Craziness: Investigating Suspected Incest* and *When
Your Child Has Been Molested: A Parents' Guide To Healing and Recovery*.

A former rape and sexual abuse treatment program director and consultant, she has been a featured expert in articles in
U.S. News and World Report, *The Washington Post*, and *Parents* magazine. In addition to her private practice, she has consulted with
and trained mental health professionals in Australia, Canada,
and throughout the United States. Together with her husband
Philip Diaz, Ms. Brohl codirects Brohl/Diaz Training and Con-
sultation in Miami.